THE
diabetes
GUIDE

CONTROL YOUR DIABETES WITH THE
COMPLETE DIET AND LIFESTYLE PLAN

Anne Claydon
Diana Markham
Graham Toms

Editor
Adam Daykin

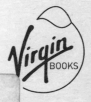

Published by Virgin Books 2009

2 4 6 8 10 9 7 5 3 1

First published in Great Britain in 2006 by
Virgin Books
Random House,
20 Vauxhall Bridge Road,
London SW1V 2SA

www.virginbooks.com
www.rbooks.co.uk

Addresses for companies within The Random House Group Limited can be found at:
www.randomhouse.co.uk/offices.htm

The Random House Group Limited Reg. No. 954009

A CIP catalogue record for this book is available from the British Library

ISBN 9780753515501

The Random House Group Limited supports The Forest Stewardship Council [FSC], the leading international forest certification organisation. All our titles that are printed on Greenpeace approved FSC certified paper carry the FSC logo.
Our paper procurement policy can be found at www.rbooks.co.uk/environment

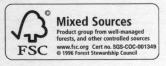

Mixed Sources
Product group from well-managed forests, and other controlled sources
www.fsc.org Cert no. SGS-COC-001349
© 1996 Forest Stewardship Council

Designed by seagulls
Printed and bound in the UK by CPI Mackays, Chatham ME5 8TD

The medical and nutritional information in this book is for reference only. The recipes and any suggestions are to be used at the reader's sole discretion and risk. Always consult a doctor if you are in doubt about nutritional or medical conditions. Never present food to anyone if it contains an ingredient that may be harmful to that person. If in doubt, ask.

contents

foreword by Sir Steve Redgrave CBE, Diabetes UK Honorary Vice-President

This book is great and a must for anybody living with diabetes. Written by diabetes professionals to provide the most credible advice, *The Diabetes Guide* not only banishes myths associated with diabetes, but also provides a comprehensive guide to living with the condition.

It is easy to forget that diabetes can be managed, but achieving this requires an understanding of the condition, and this book provides just that. *The Diabetes Guide* is clear and concise, detailing little changes that can be made to your lifestyle to lead a full and healthy life. After all, it is the little changes that make all the difference.

What I particularly love about the guide is the practical advice offered, which remains realistic, helping you to achieve better balance and control. *The Diabetes Guide* makes diabetes manageable – increased physical exercise doesn't mean you need to train for a marathon and reducing fat and sugar doesn't mean you need to lose the flavour in your food.

The Diabetes Guide is the perfect tool for anyone with diabetes who wishes to lead a full and active life whilst respecting the condition.

What an excellent way to celebrate seventy-five years of outstanding achievement from Diabetes UK by re-launching this hugely successful book!

foreword by Douglas Smallwood, CEO Diabetes UK

This is not a medical textbook, nor is it a guide to diabetes medication. It is an accessible and practical guide to living a healthy lifestyle, which is not only a cornerstone of Type 1 and Type 2 diabetes care, but also of enormous benefit to all of us. However, for people living with diabetes the benefits of a healthier lifestyle have been proven to reduce the risk of the serious complications associated with the condition; these include damage to the nerves of the hands and feet; heart attack and stroke; kidney damage and damage to the back of the eye, which can cause blindness.

Caring for your diabetes can be seen in terms of the following equation:

Good blood pressure control + good blood glucose control + weight management + increased physical activity = reduced risk of complications*

*The United Kingdom Prospective Diabetes Study 1998

This book will help you to achieve these goals by showing you how small changes in your current lifestyle can make a big difference to your wellbeing. The recipes will show you how, with small alterations, you can make substantial changes to the fat and sugar content of your favourite foods, without losing the taste. The section on physical activity will show you that you don't have to don a leotard and join a gym to increase your fitness levels. Once again little changes in your routine will reap major health benefits.

The information in this book will help you manage your diabetes more effectively, enabling you to live a full and active life.

introduction

If you have diabetes, you're certainly not alone. There are currently 2.3 million people in the UK diagnosed with the condition and more than 500,000 have Type 2 diabetes but don't know it. These figures are set to soar over the coming years, with experts predicting that by 2025 more than 4 million people in the UK and 380 million worldwide will have diabetes. It's clear that diabetes is now one of the biggest health challenges of our time.

While these figures might not make you feel a whole lot better, the truth is that healthcare professionals and scientists around the world spend a lot of time understanding how to treat and manage diabetes. And one thing is clear: by eating a healthy balanced diet, taking regular physical activity and managing your weight, you can reduce your risk of long-term complications and delay the onset of Type 2 diabetes – even preventing it in some cases.

There are a number of factors that can increase your risk of diabetes, but a leading cause of the most common form – Type 2 diabetes – is being overweight. Of course, not everyone with the condition is overweight, but the fact is that the larger your waist and the more inactive you are, the greater your risk of developing Type 2 diabetes. Perhaps most worrying of all, what was once referred to as 'late-onset diabetes', as it generally occurred in people over forty, is now being seen more often in younger people. Children and teenagers today lead increasingly sedentary lifestyles and as a result are more overweight, and therefore more prone to developing Type 2 diabetes.

While this might all sound a little alarming, the good news is that the very factors which are contributing to the rise in diabetes – namely our diet, activity levels and weight – are all within our control. And the even better news is that you don't have to drastically alter your lifestyle in order to have an effect on your health. Small, simple changes can make all the difference, and that's where this book comes in.

The Diabetes Guide offers a complete diet, physical activity and lifestyle plan with simple and realistic targets that can greatly improve your health – whether you have diabetes, you suspect you're at risk of developing it, or if you simply want to learn more about the relationship between diabetes and the virtues of a healthy lifestyle.

You don't have to go on a restrictive and punishing diet. Rather, through some simple substitutions and by adapting your favourite meals to make them healthier, you can effortlessly transform your diet and cooking habits. There are lots of great recipes in this book, many of them supplied by healthcare professionals and patients, and all of them simple and quick to make, using delicious and fresh ingredients.

Nor do you have to embark on a radical new fitness programme, or shell out a small fortune on gym membership. The worst you will have to endure, quite literally, is committing to increase whatever your chosen activity is. What a small price to pay for an insurance policy on your future health, as well as that of your family.

Even better, while making these small changes to your diet and lifestyle will certainly help you control your diabetes or help reduce your risk of developing it in the first place, these very lifestyle factors can also help stave off most of the other major Western diseases, including cancer and heart disease. In other words, you can't lose!

With the help of the authors of this book – all of them experts in the field and NHS professionals with many years' experience – you can take control of your condition and prevent diabetes from controlling you.

diabetes uncovered

WHAT IS DIABETES?

Diabetes is an increasingly common disorder. There are now more than two million people in the United Kingdom who are known to have diabetes, and around 1 million with diabetes who don't know they have it. Added to which, the number of diagnosed and undiagnosed people with diabetes is set to double over the next 10 years. If you have diabetes, in other words, there is no reason to feel isolated – you are one of many!

Diabetes occurs when the level of glucose (the main form of sugar used by the body) in your blood is too high, and your body cannot use it for energy.

> Diabetes occurs when the glucose level in your blood is too high.

HOW IS THE BLOOD GLUCOSE LEVEL CONTROLLED NORMALLY?

The pancreas is a gland situated just under the stomach. One of its functions is to produce a hormone called insulin. The insulin is produced by special cells in the pancreas called the beta cells. Insulin has the key role in promoting the uptake of glucose from the bloodstream into the muscles of the body, where it can either be used as a fuel for energy or stored for later use.

❑ **What happens when you don't have diabetes?**
When you eat a meal, some of the food is broken down into glucose by digestion in your intestine. The glucose is taken up into your bloodstream, so that it can be circulated around the body and used by your muscles.

A rise in glucose triggers the pancreas to release insulin.

Insulin allows the glucose to go from the blood into the muscles, where it is used as the main source of fuel to create energy. When the glucose has moved to your muscles, the glucose level in your blood falls to normal levels and remains steady until your next meal.

> Normally the glucose in the blood is transferred to the muscles by insulin.

❑ What happens when you have diabetes?

There are two main types of diabetes called Type 1 and Type 2 diabetes. Type 1 diabetes arises when the beta cells of your pancreas no longer produce insulin. *This is called insulin deficiency*. If you have Type 2 diabetes, your pancreas is able to produce some insulin but there is some resistance to the action of insulin which promotes the uptake of glucose into your muscles. *This is called insulin resistance*. Either way, there is a lack of glucose on the muscles and a build up of glucose in the bloodstream. The blood glucose level will rise above the normal range and will reach the point where a lot of glucose spills out into the urine, forcing the kidneys to allow more body water into the urine. You will now start to experience obvious symptoms (see below) and your urine will test positive for glucose using a simple dipstick test. It will also taste sweet!

> Diabetes develops when insufficient insulin is produced and/or the body is not able to use the insulin properly, so the glucose cannot get from the blood to the muscles.

WHAT WOULD YOU FEEL LIKE IF YOU HAD DIABETES?

If you are one of the 1 million people in the UK who have diabetes but are not aware of it, you may experience some (but not necessarily all) of the following symptoms.

❏ **Passing a lot of urine, especially at night**
Your body tries to flush the excess glucose out of your body by filtering it from the blood and passing it in your urine.

❏ **Increased thirst**
Because you are passing a lot of urine your body needs to take on more fluids to prevent dehydration.

❏ **Lethargy or loss of energy**
The glucose cannot get from the blood into the muscles. So you will feel low on energy.

❏ **Recurring infections such as thrush, urine infections or boils**
High levels of glucose in the blood are a good source of food for bacteria and fungi, and your immune system becomes compromised.

❏ **Temporary blurred vision**
High glucose levels in the blood temporarily affect glucose content in the fluid compartments of your eyes, causing blurred vision. This is usually temporary – once diabetes is under control, your vision may return to normal.

❏ **Weight loss**
Weight loss occurs principally in people with Type1 diabetes, but may occur also with Type 2 diabetes.

If you think you have some of these symptoms, it is recommended that you see your GP who will perform a simple blood test which will tell if you have diabetes or not.

There are two main types of diabetes: Type 1 and Type 2. Type 2 is far more common than Type 1.

TYPES OF DIABETES

There are two types of diabetes: Type 1 and Type 2.

Type 1 diabetes usually develops quickly over a few weeks and predominantly affects children and young adults. People with Type 1 diabetes produce very little or no insulin and must manage their condition with insulin injections.

Type 2 diabetes usually develops in people over the age of 40, but increasingly it is developing at a younger age. It develops slowly and many people don't realise they have it, as symptoms do not usually appear for many years. You may simply feel more tired than usual and many put this down to working too hard or getting older. People with Type 2 diabetes still produce insulin but either not enough, or the amount they do produce may not work properly. They do not necessarily need to inject insulin – they can often treat their diabetes with diet and excerise alone or in combination with tablets.

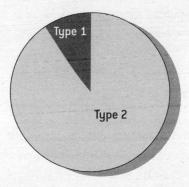

In 2004 there were approximately 237,000 people in the UK with Type 1 diabetes and 1.53 million with Type 2 diabetes.

❑ **Type 1 diabetes is treated by:**
- Insulin injections
- Healthy eating
- Regular exercise

❑ **Type 2 diabetes is treated by:**
- Healthy eating
- Regular exercise
- Tablets, possibly leading to insulin

> Type 1 diabetes usually develops over a few weeks and predominantly affects children and young adults. Type 2 diabetes develops slowly so that people often don't recognise they have it. It usually occurs in people over 40, but can occur in much younger people.

WHY DO SOME PEOPLE GET DIABETES AND NOT OTHERS?

❑ **Type 1 diabetes**

In Type 1 diabetes the insulin-producing cells of the pancreas are destroyed by a malfunction of the immune system, possibly triggered by a viral infection. The exact mechanism for developing this disease is not fully understood, but is the subject of much scientific research worldwide.

❑ **Type 2 diabetes**

In Type 2 diabetes there is still some insulin produced by the pancreas, but not enough and what is produced may not work very well. Being overweight is the main cause of Type 2 diabetes. People who are particularly at risk have a large amount of fat, known as intra-abdominal fat, contained within their abdominal cavity – they are typically 'apple-shaped'. Over time, as the potential Type 2 diabetic continues to build up intra-abdominal fat, the insulin

The following factors make you more susceptible to developing Type 2 diabetes:
- Being overweight
- Lack of physical activity
- Having a family history of diabetes
- Being of South Asian, African or Caribbean ethnicity
- Having had diabetes during pregnancy

producing cells are worked harder and harder and the insulin becomes less effective. This is the point at which the *potential* Type 2 diabetic becomes an *actual* Type 2 diabetic, with all its implications. Although the diabetes is unlikely to be reversed, the situation can be improved by simply losing weight. Remember, it's the intra-abdominal fat which causes insulin to be used less effectively. It makes sense – lose some of that intra-abdominal fat and the insulin will be used more effectively. If weight gain in adults were prevented most of all Type 2 diabetes would be eliminated.

Type 2 diabetes was called 'maturity onset diabetes', as it usually occurs in the over 40s. However, today we are seeing younger and younger people with this type of diabetes. The reasons for this are obvious – obese people are far more prone to this type of diabetes and, sadly, teenagers today are increasingly overweight, as a result of their 'couch potato' lifestyle.

Type 2 diabetes can also run in the family, so diabetes sufferers should make an effort to get their children involved in their new health regimen. If you're of South Asian, African or Caribbean ethnicity, there is also an increased chance that you have the genetic predisposition to the disease.

OTHER CAUSES OF DIABETES

❑ **Prescribed Medication**

Some medication prescribed by your doctor may increase your blood sugar. Drugs such as steroids may bring about a temporary increase in blood sugar or may reveal diabetes that you have actually had for a while.

❑ **Diseases of the pancreas**

If you develop an illness such as pancreatitis, diabetes may develop. If your pancreas has to be removed surgically due to illness, you will develop diabetes.

❑ **Serious illness**

During a heart attack, or if you are in hospital having surgery, your blood sugar may rise and bring about a temporary form of diabetes.

❑ **Pregnancy**

Diabetes may develop during pregnancy. This is known as gestational diabetes. It usually resolves itself after pregnancy and does not result in the baby also getting the disease. Mothers with this condition may be more prone to diabetes later in life, so it's a good idea to follow a healthy lifestyle.

> Being overweight and physically inactive are the major causes of Type 2 diabetes in people who have the genetic predisposition for the condition.

HISTORICAL BACKGROUND

You'd be forgiven for thinking that diabetes is a relatively new disease as it's only over the last 50 or so years that it's become a major global healthcare priority. In reality, diabetes has been around for at least 3,000 years. The first known records of a diabetes-like condition are found in ancient manuscripts uncovered in Asia Minor and Egypt. At the time, the disease had not been named, so manuscripts talked only of the condition's distinctive symptoms: boils and infections, excessive thirst, loss of weight and, bizarrely, sweet-tasting urine.

(Sweet urine was a useful symptom, since it made for an effective means of diagnosis – for many years, doctors identified patients with diabetes by dipping their finger into their urine and tasting it! Today your doctor will administer a far more hygienic blood test.) In 1776, a young physician practising at the Liverpool Public Infirmary called Matthew Dobson made the important connection of sugar passing from blood to kidneys to urine. Dobson recognised that diabetes occurs when blood sugar, or glucose, is too high. At the time physicians were also establishing the link between blood sugar and food. That is, you eat; your body digests the food you've just eaten; blood sugar levels rise. However, knowledge about the precise link between food and diabetes was sketchy, to say the least. Two schools of thought developed. In the late 1850s, French doctor Priorry advised his diabetes patients to eat extra sugar to replace the amount lost in the urine – not the brightest of ideas! Bouchardat, another Frenchman, developed another school of thought, advocating an extremely low calorie diet, essentially starving the patient. Again, not ideal.

Luckily, our understanding of how food, and more generally, lifestyle affects diabetes has improved substantially over the last 150 years. We are now at a stage where we can provide clinically proven advice about the ways in which healthy eating and lifestyle

The word diabetes was first used around the 2nd century BC. The full name given to the condition was diabetes mellitus (diabetes is a Greek word meaning siphon or fountain; mellitus is Latin for sweetness). Literally translated, it means 'sweet-tasting urine'.

can improve the quality of life of those with diabetes, as well as reducing the risk of the full blown disease from developing in the first place.

POPULAR MYTHS ABOUT DEVELOPING DIABETES

Everybody knows somebody with diabetes and, inevitably, there are many myths about the illness floating around. For example, that 'one chocolate bar too many' brings about the disease. You do not develop diabetes by taking too much sugar, although if you do over-indulge in high calorie foods in general, you may develop diabetes through being overweight. Similarly, you can't 'catch diabetes from somebody else', and being 'stressed out' or the 'soggy British weather' have absolutely nothing to do with whether you have diabetes or not!

There is no such thing as 'mild diabetes'. Until relatively recent times, people diagnosed as having Type 2 diabetes might have been told by health professionals that they had a 'mild' form of diabetes as the symptoms of the condition could often be controlled by dietary treatment alone, in contrast to Type 1 diabetes which could be life threatening at diagnosis unless insulin treatment was started straightaway.

During the past few years, we have come to learn that Type 2 diabetes is a far more serious condition than originally thought due to its genetic link to other risk factors (e.g. high blood pressure and cholesterol) for cardiovascular disease such as coronary heart disease and stroke. People with Type 2 diabetes have a threefold increased risk of suffering a heart attack compared to the general population, and this is the commonest cause of premature death in people who have the disease.

COMPLICATIONS OF DIABETES

A good management of diabetes is absolutely paramount. A number of longer-term health problems arise when blood sugar levels remain high for a prolonged period. When blood glucose remains high the blood becomes a little more sticky and has difficulty flowing through the veins and arteries. This may lead to a whole range of long-term blood circulation problems. For example, damage to blood vessels results in an increased chance of strokes and heart attacks. People with diabetes are particularly prone to blood vessels becoming clogged up, or furring up with deposits of fat, know as cholesterol. Additionally, when there is a large amount of glucose in the blood, nerves can become damaged which can lead to a loss of sensation in the feet. You are less likely to feel a cut or graze and your feet become susceptible to infection due to the high levels of blood glucose (glucose acts as a good food source for bacteria). Diabetes can also lead to a blurring of the vision, while impotence sometimes occurs in men due to circulatory and nerve damage problems.

Hypoglycaemia is a common complication of diabetes. It occurs when blood sugar levels are too low. The condition affects people who take insulin or certain tablets to treat their diabetes. There are a number of reasons why you might become hypoglycaemic, or have a 'hypo'. These are:

- You missed a meal or snack.
- You're eating too little or dieting.
- You've done more physical exercise than usual.
- You've taken too much insulin or too many diabetes tablets.
- You've drunk alcohol without food.
- The weather is very hot.

It is proven that if you keep your blood sugar under control, there is less chance of developing these complications. However, with the best will in the world, some complications may develop over the years, purely down to the long term damaging nature of diabetes.

Diabetic complications usually affect the eyes, kidneys, nerves, legs and small blood vessels. Treating secondary complications is a huge drain on NHS resources and has a drastic knock-on effect on the British economy. Diabetes treatment currently accounts for an incredible 9% of the total NHS spend on healthcare – that's approximately £5 billion per annum. Of this, around £2 billion is spent on treating secondary complications, which often only occur through poor management of diabetes and are therefore completely avoidable.

❑ Eyes

Diabetic retinopathy affects the eyes. Diabetic retinopathy is damage of the small blood vessels at the back of the eye.

There are two types of damage:

- *Background retinopathy* is when the blood vessels in the retina (where images are formed at the back of the eye) develop tiny bulges which leak fluid and form deposits. Mild background retinopathy is usually not treated and people do not develop symptoms.
- *Proliferate retinopathy* occurs when new blood vessels on the retina rupture and bleed into the fluid chamber of the eye called the vitreous, causing blocking of light from the retina. This leakage of blood can lead to the formation of scar tissue within the vitreous and can lead to detachment of the retina. Proliferate retinopathy is treated by laser.

To cut down on the risk of developing diabetes retinopathy:
- Keep your blood sugar under control.
- Maintain normal blood pressure – get it checked regularly by your healthcare team.
- Have your eyes examined yearly by a digital camera (ask your practice nurse or doctor about this).

❑ The Kidneys

The kidneys filter waste products from the blood, take away excess water and expel certain chemicals. Diabetes can lead to damage to the kidneys called diabetic nephropathy.

Diabetic nephropathy usually develops slowly over many years. Kidney filtering becomes insufficient and proteins leak out into the urine. Your doctor will check your urine for protein yearly. Other symptoms are high blood pressure, fluid retention and fatigue. When the damage to the kidneys becomes very advanced, treatment with dialysis becomes necessary. Kidney transplant is another option if available.

> To cut down on the risk of diabetes nephropathy:
> - Keep blood glucose well controlled.
> - Maintain good blood pressure – get it regularly checked.
> - You may need a special diet.

❑ Nerve damage

Nerve damage is called neuropathy. It occurs in both Type 1 and Type 2 diabetes. Constant high blood glucose damages the nerves and this results in the loss of sensation and pain.

Peripheral neuropathy causes changes in sensation that starts in the toes and spreads to the feet and legs. The patient complains of numbness, tingling, burning or cramp. This is usually worse at night.

The biggest problem with peripheral neuropathy is that people develop foot ulcers. As they do not feel pain they may inadvertently stand on a sharp object or blister their feet in new shoes and injure themselves and not be aware of it leaving time before the ulcer is discovered.

> To cut down on the risk of peripheral neuropathy:
> - Keep blood glucose under control.
> - Check your feet daily.
> - See your podiatrist at least annually.

☐ Disease of blood vessels

Macrovascular disease refers to changes to the medium to large size blood vessels. The vessel walls become thickened and non-elastic. Plaque, a deposit, also develops and the vessels may become blocked.

There are three types of this disease:

- *Peripheral Vascular Disease* refers to blood vessels that supply the legs and feet. If the vessel is partially blocked, cramps and pain on walking may develop. A complete blockage will produce severe pain and the leg will become cold – no pulse can be felt. Urgent hospital treatment is required and it may be possible to unblock or bypass the diseased artery.

- *Coronary Artery Disease* refers to diseased arteries in the heart. Complete blockage of an artery results in a heart attack (myocardial infarction). Symptoms of a heart attack or angina include a heavy feeling in the chest, shortness of breath and chest pain. However, due to nerve damage some people with diabetes may feel no pain in the chest and suffer a so-called 'silent myocardial infarction'. People suffering a suspected heart attack need emergency hospital treatment which may lead to a procedure to unblock the diseased coronary artery (coronary angioplasty) or a coronary artery bypass graft (CABG) operation.

How to cut down the risk of arterial disease:

- Keep blood sugar well controlled.
- Maintain good blood pressure – see your doctor and get it checked.
- If overweight, try to reduce it.
- Reduce fats in your diet.
- Do not smoke.
- Know your cholesterol level – your doctor will prescribe medication to help lower it if necessary.
- Exercise for 30 mins at least 4 times a week.

- *Cerebro-vascular Disease* is when there is a damaged artery in the brain. This may result in a stroke. Symptoms include: drowsiness, headaches, loss of ability to speak, paralysis of one side of the body.

THE FUTURE OF DIABETES

Statistics speak for themselves: the prevalence of Type 2 diabetes is set to increase from its present level of 150 million worldwide to 220 million by the end of the decade, and to 300 million by 2025. In the UK alone the number of people with Type 2 diabetes is predicted to reach 3 million by 2010. That means another 1.2 million people in the UK with Type 2 diabetes over the next five years. The reason for this rapid increase is linked to the way in which people of all cultures have embraced the Western lifestyle.

If you are overweight and do little exercise and if you have a family history of diabetes, it is possible that one of these newly diagnosed people will be you. Plus, if you have Type 2 diabetes and you have children, they may also be at risk. Consider the recent statistics. In 2004 the World Health Organisation (WHO) estimated that 10% of school-aged children were overweight and that Type 2 diabetes will increase in this age group. In a recent study in East London it was shown that 10% of children below the age of 16 and 34% of young people between the age of 16 and 25 years with diabetes had Type 2 diabetes. All the children and young people with Type 2 diabetes were obese (BMI at least 30).

Thankfully, this situation is actually easy to remedy. And it takes very little effort. This book will help you to simply modify your diet and lifestyle with the help of easy recipes and tips on exercise – read on and you're halfway there already.

SUMMARY: DIABETES UNCOVERED

- Diabetes occurs when the glucose level in your blood is too high.
- In normal cases, glucose is transferred to the muscles by insulin.
- Diabetes develops when not enough insulin is produced and/or the body does not use the insulin sufficiently, so that the glucose cannot get from the blood to the muscles.
- There are two main types of diabetes: Type 1 and Type 2. Type 2 is far more common than Type 1.
- Type 1 usually develops over a few weeks and predominantly affects children and young adults. Type 2 diabetes develops slowly so that people often do not recognise they have it. It usually occurs in people over 40, but can occur in much younger people.
- Being overweight and physically inactive are the major causes of Type 2 diabetes.
- There could be approximately 1.2 million people diagnosed with Type 2 diabetes over the next five years. Modification to diet and activity is the key to reducing this number and helping those with the disease.

the diabetes principles

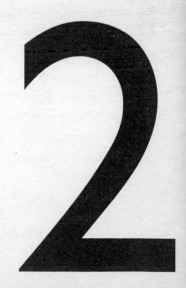

healthy eating

by Diana Markham, Chief Dietitian, Newham University Hospital NHS Trust

INTRODUCTION

Food plays an important part in all our lives. But it doesn't take a dietitian to tell us that its importance extends way beyond the need to survive. The daily decisions we make about the food we eat affect our health and well-being directly. The expression 'you are what you eat' is certainly an accurate one!

Many of the major healthcare conditions are affected by diet, diabetes being a prime example. As an experienced NHS dietitian, I have seen a steady increase over the years in the number of people developing Type 2 diabetes. There is no doubt that bad eating habits are one of the prime reasons for this. The good news is that along with advances in understanding how the wrong diet can affect the condition, we also know how the right diet can improve it.

Many of my patients have found creative, exciting ways to adapt their favourite recipes, and they are already feeling better as a result of it. Our recipe section shows ways to make traditional recipes healthier just by adapting cooking methods (opting for grilling or baking rather than frying), and reducing the amount of fat, salt and sugar we use. There's no need to jettison all of your eating and cooking habits! Flavour need not be compromised, either – dishes will taste just as good, if not better, when prepared with healthy ingredients. And remember, healthy cooking and eating is good for one and all, not just those who suffer from diabetes. You'll be surprised how quickly it will become part of your everyday life.

For people with diabetes, your treatment may be by diet alone, tablets or insulin therapy. Whatever treatment you are prescribed, you should still follow a good diet.

THE EIGHT GUIDING PRINCIPLES

If you have diabetes or are at risk of developing it, the following main Guiding Principles will help you to adapt and improve your diet.

1. **Eat regular meals**
2. **Include a variety of foods from the four main food groups**
3. **Eat fewer sugary foods**
4. **Eat less fried and fatty foods**
5. **Include more low GI foods**
6. **Reduce your salt intake**
7. **Go easy with alcohol**
8. **Avoid special 'diabetic' products**

Following a healthy diet also helps to reduce the risk of becoming overweight and of developing heart disease. A healthy diet benefits everybody – not just people with diabetes.

1. EAT REGULAR MEALS

Getting three meals a day (breakfast, lunch and dinner) will go some way towards keeping your diet varied. This is critical for people with diabetes, as it will help keep blood sugar levels steady, which in turn means you won't feel so hungry and you'll have more energy. You'll also avoid getting caught in a high blood sugar/low blood sugar cycle which makes you prone to overeating.

2. INCLUDE A VARIETY OF FOODS FROM THE FOUR MAIN FOOD GROUPS

The main nutrients are carbohydrates, proteins and fats. Micro nutrients, which are vitamins, minerals and trace elements, are also essential for good health. See the chart below as a guide to a balanced combination of foods.

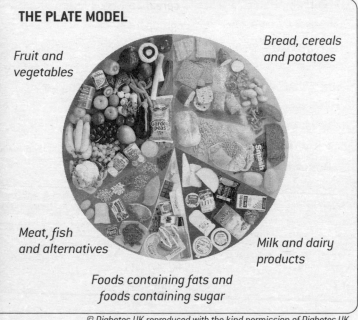

THE PLATE MODEL

Fruit and vegetables

Bread, cereals and potatoes

Meat, fish and alternatives

Milk and dairy products

Foods containing fats and foods containing sugar

© Diabetes UK reproduced with the kind permission of Diabetes UK.

❏ **Fruit and vegetables**

Provide fibre, and are good sources of vitamin C and anti-oxidants, which have protective health benefits. Select fresh, frozen, dried and tinned products. Tinned fruit should be canned in natural juice or water rather than syrup. The recommendations are that we should include at least five servings of fruits and vegetables a day. As some fruit natually contains quite a lot of sugar we would advise people with diabetes to limit their intake to one or two portions at a time in order to keep blood sugar levels within the optimal range.

A commonly asked question is: 'What constitutes a portion of fruit?'

The answer is: 1 medium-sized apple, orange or pear; 1 small banana; 10 grapes; 2 apricots; 1 peach or nectarine; 1 slice of melon or 2 kiwi fruits.

❑ **Carbohydrates (e.g. bread, cereal and potatoes)**
Our main source of energy. This group includes both starches and sugars. As a general rule, starches are better than sugars for keeping blood sugar levels steady – try to include something from the group of starchy foods at each meal.

❑ **Meat, fish and alternatives**
These foods are all good sources of protein which is essential for good health. Examples include red meat, chicken, fish, eggs, soya, beans and lentils. Include two servings per day.

❑ **Milk and dairy foods**
These are good sources of protein and calcium, which is important for strong bones. Examples include milk, yoghurt, fromage frais and cheese. Include two servings per day and select low fat varieties e.g. semi-skimmed milk, low fat or 'diet' yoghurts, low fat cheeses like cottage cheese or reduced fat cheddar.

3. EAT FEWER SUGARY FOODS

As well as raising your blood sugar levels rapidly, sugary foods are often high in calories and lack nutritional value – so are best avoided. However if you really can't imagine foregoing sweet things altogether, use artificial sweetener instead of sugar, particularly in tea and coffee and on cereals. Select 'no added sugar' squashes and 'diet' soft drinks. Try to limit your intake of desserts and confectionery. Your taste buds adapt to less sugar over a period of around three weeks, so it does become easier.

4. EAT LESS FRIED AND FATTY FOOD

Fat in equals fat on! It's not rocket science – if you regularly eat a large amount of fried or fatty food you will put on weight. Additionally if you are eating saturated fats like fatty meat, cream, full fat milk, cheese, butter and ghee, and some vegetable fats like palm oil and coconut cream, your cholesterol level will rise accordingly.

> Cholesterol is a waxy substance which sticks to the walls of arteries, restricting the flow of blood. It is a major cause of heart disease. People with diabetes are particularly prone to heart disease because high glucose levels thicken up the blood, restricting its flow.

The good news is that most dishes can be made using less oil. As a guide, a tablespoon of oil is quite enough for a dish that serves 4–6 people. Use oils that are better for you, like monounsaturated oil (e.g. olive oil and spread) or polyunsaturated oils and spreads (e.g. sunflower and corn oils and spreads), both in cooking and for spreading on bread.

> Saturated fats are usually hard at room temperature.

5. INCLUDE MORE LOW-GI FOODS

Foods containing carbohydrates have different effects on your blood sugar levels. This response is called the glycaemic index (GI). Foods that raise blood sugar levels slowly have a low GI, while foods that raise blood sugar levels quickly have a high GI. In other words, low GI foods are good for keeping blood sugar levels stable, which is excellent news for people with diabetes, not to mention the fact that they also make you feel fuller for longer. As a general rule, try to include at least one low GI food at each meal. It's easy to start making a difference!

6. REDUCE YOUR SALT INTAKE

If your diet includes a lot of salt, there is more chance that you will develop high blood pressure. Since people with diabetes are up to twice as likely to have high blood pressure anyway, reducing salt intake is a good idea. Use just a little salt in cooking if you must, but don't add any when you're at the table. Use pepper, herbs and spices to flavour your dishes instead. The recommended daily amount of salt is 6g.

7. GO EASY WITH ALCOHOL

A high alcohol intake can result in hypoglycaemia, your blood sugar dropping too low. This is because alcohol reduces the rate of glucose conversion in the liver. For people with diabetes, especially those on insulin therapy, this can lead to hypoglycaemia. If you must have a drink, be very moderate, spreading your allowed units evenly over the week – don't binge drink, whatever you do. Try to have two alcohol free days each week.

8. AVOID SPECIAL 'DIABETIC' PRODUCTS

Special 'diabetic' products have no particular benefits. They are expensive to buy, they don't taste as good as regular alternatives and the sweetening agent sometimes used (sorbitol) has a laxative effect. Opt instead for products from your local supermarket which have a reduced sugar and fat content.

WHAT IS FOOD MADE UP OF?

Food is made up of different components and these are explained here in detail.

CARBOHYDRATES

Carbohydrates are either starches or sugars and they are the main sources of energy for your body. Interestingly, they are all of vegetable origin.

❑ **Starch**
Starchy foods are broken down relatively slowly into glucose in the body, so they keep the blood sugar levels fairly steady. Examples of foods in this group include rice, bread, pulses, other flour-based products such as chapattis, pasta, potatoes, plantain, yam and breakfast cereals. Starchy foods should be included with each main meal of the day and may also be included as snacks between meals for people with diabetes.

> If you have diabetes, go for moderate portion sizes of starchy foods to keep blood glucose levels nice and steady.

❑ **Sugar**
Sugar raises blood sugar levels quite quickly so intake should be limited. It's sensible to avoid adding sugar to drinks and breakfast cereals and use low sugar options where possible. If you want to sweeten beverages and foods, then use an artificial sweetener of which there are many varieties available in both tablet and powdered form. Examples currently available include Canderel, Hermasetas, Splenda, saccharin and supermarket own brands. Many different soft drinks have artificial sweetening agents instead of sugar, and are identified

by the labelling 'no added sugar' (for squashes) and 'diet' for fizzy drinks.

Desserts should be limited as they usually have a high sugar, and often fat, content. Select lower sugar and fat options. 'Regular' desserts should be kept for special occasions. Even then, go easy on portion sizes!

Confectionery should be limited to small amounts only, and it is best to include such items after a meal rather than in between. This is because the bulk of the food you have eaten at the meal will slow down the rate of absorption of the sugar into your bloodstream.

PROTEIN

Protein is vital for the structure and function of your body. It's a major component of body tissues and is therefore essential for the growth and maintenance of body tissue throughout your life. Additionally proteins can also be used to provide energy, if carbohydrate sources are inadequate. Proteins also have other roles in your body which include some enzyme, hormone, and immune functions. Animal protein sources include meat, poultry, fish, eggs and dairy products, such as milk, cheese and yoghurt. Keep meat

There are 20 amino acids which are incorporated into protein, of which 9 are termed 'essential', as the human body cannot synthesize these and they must therefore be provided in our diets. Choosing a variety of different protein-containing foods in your diet ensures that you obtain a variety of different amino acids, which your body can then use as required. Surplus amino acids are converted to urea and excreted by the kidneys – some of this surplus is converted to glucose and can be used as a source of energy.

and poultry cuts lean and include fish at least twice a week, with one portion being oily fish. Make sure the dairy products you go for are low fat varieties. Vegetable sources include pulses, such as lentils, beans and peas, cereals and nuts. If you are vegetarian, these foods are particularly important sources of protein.

> **Enzyme** – A protein produced by living organisms that promotes or otherwise influences chemical reactions.
>
> **Hormone** – A protein that is made by one part of the body but affects another part of the body.
>
> **Immune function** – Production and action of cells that fight disease or infection.

FATS AND OILS

Fat is present in every cell in your body and has a wide range of roles. Fat is a component of brain tissue and cells. Fat provides a protective layer around essential organs like the kidneys. It also insulates the body against heat loss. Fat is also a source of fuel and a reserve energy supply.

We also need some fat in our diet to make sure we get the essential fatty acids that our bodies cannot produce and the fat-soluble vitamins A, D & E. A small amount of fat also makes food palatable.

Fats and oils contain the greatest amount of energy in your diet, so a diet high in fat will contribute to weight gain. Regardless of their source, fats and oils all have the same energy content per gram/ml/fluid ounce. To distinguish between them: fats are solid at room temperature e.g. butter, ghee, margarine, the fat on meat, while oils are liquid at room temperature e.g. olive, sunflower and corn oils.

Dietary fats are made up of different fatty acids. There are 21 of these fatty acids found in our diet. The two essential fatty acids that the body cannot produce are linoleic acid and alpha-linolenic acid.

There are two types of fats: saturated (including trans fats) and unsaturated which are polyunsaturated and monounsaturated fats.

❑ Saturated fats

Saturated fats are solid at room temperature. They have a particularly detrimental effect on your health, since they raise cholesterol levels, and high cholesterol levels mean a greater risk of developing heart disease.

Sources of saturated fats are:
- Meat and meat products;
- Full fat milk, cheeses and yoghurts, cream, butter;
- Coconut oil and cream, palm oil;
- Baked products like biscuits, cakes, pastries and chocolate.

Cholesterol is a waxy substance which is necessary in modest amounts in the body. It is a component of cell membranes, present in some enzyme systems and is required in the synthesis of bile and vitamin D.

There are two types of cholesterol:
- GOOD! High-density lipoprotein (HDL) that removes excess cholesterol from the blood and takes it to the liver for disposal. Another beneficial effect of regular exercise is that it raises HDL levels.
- BAD! Low-density lipoprotein (LDL) that can be deposited on the artery walls, narrowing them and thus increasing the risk of heart attack.

Two thirds of our cholesterol is produced by the liver, and around one third comes from dietary sources. This is why dietary cholesterol has only a small effect on our blood cholesterol levels.

Many adults have cholesterol levels higher than they should be, partly as a result of dietary and lifestyle habits. Your GP can arrange a blood test to check out your cholesterol level. People with diabetes are more likely to have raised cholesterol levels as a direct result of changes in their bodies due to their condition. Medication such as statins is usually prescribed to people with high cholesterol. The current guidance for the normal range of total cholesterol is 4.0 mmol/litre or less for a person with diabetes.

Reduce the intake of foods with a high cholesterol content like liver, offal, pâté and products made with shellfish, fish roe and egg yolks. If your cholesterol level is high, limit your intake of these foods to a maximum of once a fortnight for offal and shellfish, and eggs to a maximum of five per week.

❑ Trans fats

Transaturated fatty acids, or trans fats, are only present naturally in very small amounts and are found in milk, cheese, beef and lamb. However, the main sources in your diets are in manufactured margarines where liquid vegetable oils are hydrogenated to make them more solid. Trans fats can be regarded as the same as saturated fats in terms of the effect that they have on our bodies. Trans fats are used a lot in manufactured food products, like cakes and biscuits.

❑ Unsaturated fats

Unsaturated fats/oils do not have the same cholesterol-raising properties as saturated fats and should be used wherever possible, for example as spreading fats, in baked products and in cooking. In fact, unsaturated fats are an important part of our diet – in limited amounts, of course. There are two types of unsaturated fat: polyunsaturated and monounsaturated.

> Cut down on your fat intake by eating fewer fried foods, reducing the amount of oil used when making dishes, using smaller amounts of spreading fats and watching out for hidden fats in manufactured foods like biscuits and snacks.

❑ Polyunsaturated fats

Polyunsaturated fats are important for many of the body's processes. They are also used as a component of the membrane structures in our bodies.

There are two types of polyunsaturated fatty acids: omega 6 and omega 3 fatty acids. Sources of omega 6 are sunflower, corn and evening primrose oils. Omega 6 lowers total cholesterol levels, but consuming excessive omega 6 is not encouraged as this may have potentially adverse effects on the body. Sources of omega 3 are fish oils, soya and rapeseed oils. Omega 3 has properties which protect against heart attacks and help the body's inflammatory response. We need a combination of both omega 3 and omega 6 fatty acids to remain healthy.

❑ Monounsaturated fats

Monounsaturated fats have a particularly beneficial effect on cholesterol levels because they lower the 'bad' LDL cholesterol without lowering the 'good' HDL cholesterol. The main dietary sources are olive and rapeseed oils. They are present as the main fat in nuts and seeds and in modest amounts in animal fats.

> Substitute saturated fats in your diet with monounsaturated oils as much as possible.

DIETARY FIBRE

Dietary fibre is the term given to complex carbohydrates that resist digestion in the human gut. Fibre is a mixture of components of plant cell walls and provides bulk in the diet. This in turn helps to maintain good bowel function.

There are two types of fibre: soluble fibre and insoluble fibre that act in different ways with the body.

❏ Soluble fibre

Soluble fibre reduces the rate at which glucose enters the bloodstream following a meal, which is particularly beneficial to people with diabetes. It helps to generate a more level blood glucose profile. Soluble fibre also reduces the total blood cholesterol levels, specifically the 'bad' LDL cholesterol. Sources of soluble fibre include fruits, vegetables, oats and lentils.

❏ Insoluble fibre

Insoluble fibre provides bulk (in this case, food which is eaten but not digested) to the intestine during digestion, helping the food move through the gut more efficiently. Additionally, some parts of the fibre have a beneficial influence on the bacteria in the large intestine and fatty acids produced as a result of bacterial fermentation. This may contribute to reducing the risk of developing colorectal cancer. Insoluble fibre is found in vegetables, fruits, wholegrain cereals, nuts and seeds.

Increase your fibre intake by making sure you eat:

- Unrefined cereal products, e.g. wholegrain options
- Pulses
- Fruit and veg (aim to meet the 'Five a Day' guidance for portions)
- Nuts and seeds

VITAMINS

Vitamins represent a wide range of substances which are essential for many of the body's processes. They are only required in very small quantities. For the majority of vitamins, dietary sources are required as the body cannot synthesize them.

Vitamin/Dietary Source

Vitamin A Meat and meat products, particularly liver, milk/dairy products and fortified margarines.

Vitamin D Fortified margarines and spreads, cereals and oily fish.

Vitamin E Margarines and spreads, particularly those that have been fortified and products where fat is a major ingredient. Wheat germ oil and sunflower seed oil.

Vitamin K Green leafy vegetables, soybean oil and beef liver.

Vitamin B1 Breakfast cereals, particularly fortified varieties, vegetables, bread and meat products. All flours in the UK, with the exception of wholemeal, are fortified with Vitamin B1.

Vitamin B2 Milk/dairy products, meat and meat products, and cereal products.

Vitamin B3 Meat and meat products, cereal products, vegetable products and milk/dairy products.

Vitamin B6 Cereals, meat and meat products, potatoes and milk/dairy products. Also present in nuts and pulses.

Vitamin B12 Animal food sources, such as meat, dairy products, fish and eggs. Small amounts are present in fortified foods like breakfast cereal.

Pantothenic Acid Yeast, offal, peanuts, meat, eggs and green vegetables.

Biotin Cereal products, beverages, milk/dairy products, eggs and meat.

Folate/Folic acid Cereal products, vegetables, milk/dairy products and meat products. Many breakfast cereals are also fortified with folate.

Vitamin C Fruits, fruit juices and vegetables.

MINERALS AND TRACE ELEMENTS

Minerals and trace elements are required in even smaller amounts than vitamins, but like vitamins, they are essential. They play a role in the following: tissue structure, enzyme systems, fluid balance, cellular function and neurotransmission.

Mineral/Dietary Source

Calcium Milk, other dairy products, such as cheese, yoghurt and fromage frais, fish containing soft bones, green leafy vegetables, pulses and tap water.

Phosphorous Milk and dairy products, cereals, meat and meat products and vegetables.

Magnesium Bread and cereal products, beverages, vegetables and potatoes, milk/dairy products.

Sodium Table salt, bread and cereals, meat and meat products (particularly ham and bacon), milk and dairy products (especially cheese), salted foods like crisps, nuts, salted biscuits and savoury snacks, and bottled sources, stock cubes etc. Canned products, packaged soups and ready meals are all significant sources of sodium.

Potassium Vegetables, fruits, beverages, especially coffee, milk and dairy products and cereal products.

Iron Red meat, offal, poultry and fish, cereals fortified with iron, white flour, which is fortified, green leafy vegetables, pulses, dried fruit, nuts and seeds.

Zinc Meat and meat products, cereals and milk/diary products.

Copper Meat, cereals, vegetables and beverages, tea and coffee.

Chromium Yeast, meat, wholegrains, legumes and nuts.

Manganese Tea is the primary source of manganese in our diets.

Selenium Meats, fish, fats, vegetables and cereals.

Fluorine Water.

FLUIDS

About 75% of our body weight is made up of water. We continually lose water from the body through urination and perspiration. Water also helps the digestion and absorption of food and is important for normal bowel function. It is essential to drink plenty of fluids throughout the day.

> As a guide, try to drink 6–8 glasses/cups of fluids each day, which is the equivalent of 1.5–2 litres of fluids. If the weather is hot or you are particularly active, you will need an even greater fluid intake.

If you don't drink enough fluids, you may become dehydrated. Signs of dehydration are extreme thirst, headache and urine which is more concentrated and darker in colour.

☐ Suitable drinks

For people with diabetes, water, teas, coffee and artificially sweetened soft drinks are all suitable.

- *Water:* Tap water or mineral water, natural or flavoured, are all great options. Chilled water is a particularly refreshing way of meeting those daily fluid requirements.
- *Squashes:* The 'no added sugar' and 'sugar free' varieties are all suitable. Examples include Robinsons 'Special R', Kia Ora 'Low Calorie' and supermarket own brands.

> Drinks labelled 'light' may not be suitable – check the label first. Go for drinks that have a maximum of 2 grams of carbohydrate per 100 ml.

- *Fizzy drinks:* Choose drinks labelled 'diet' and 'low calorie'. Examples include Diet Coke, Diet Pepsi, Light 7-Up, Lucozade Lo-cal, Slimline mixers.
- *Carton and juice drinks:* Choose drinks labelled 'no added sugar' or 'sugar free'. Examples include Ribena 'no added sugar' and Robinsons 'no added sugar'.

> Drinks that contain small amounts of natural sugar should be limited. They may have more than 2 grams of carbohydrate per 100 ml. Avoid drinks that are sweetened with added sugar. Check the Nutrition Information box on drinks if you are unsure whether they are suitable or not.

- *Hot drinks:* Black teas, green teas, herbal and fruit teas and coffees are all suitable. If necessary, use an artificial sweetener.
- *Milk and fruit juices:* Milk and fruit juices contain small amounts of natural sugar, so contain more calories than sugar free drinks. Drink these in modest amounts to avoid rising blood sugar levels.

> Limit your intake of milk and fruit juices as they contain natural sugar.
> **Milk:** we advise that you limit quantities to a glass (200 ml or ⅓ pint) at a time and choose lower fat milk
> **Fruit juice:** 100 ml glass (small glass) – 1–2 glasses per day

❑ Alcoholic drinks

You may drink alcohol in limited amounts. Men should aim to keep their intake below 21 units per week (2–3 units per day) and women below 14 units per week (1–2 units per day), with 2 alcohol-free days each week. Go easy, in other words.

Six Rules to remember when having alcoholic drinks:

1. Never drink on an empty stomach as alcohol can lower your blood sugar level. (For people with diabetes, this could lead to hypoglycaemia.)
2. If you're drinking alcohol in the evening, remember to have a snack before bedtime such as toast, a glass of milk or two plain biscuits/crackers.
3. All alcoholic drinks are high in calories and may lead to weight gain.
4. 'Diabetic' beers and lagers are higher in alcohol than normal varieties (as well as being expensive), and are best avoided.
5. 'Alco-pops' should be avoided as they are high in sugar.
6. Choose low calorie or 'diet' mixers to accompany spirits.

> One unit of alcohol =
> ½ pint of beer/lager/bitter/cider
> 1 small glass of wine (125 ml)
> 1 single 'pub' measure of spirits (25 ml)
>
> Take care as some beers, lagers and ciders have a higher alcoholic content than standard brands so a measure of these drinks will contain more than one unit of alcohol.

GLYCAEMIC INDEX

The Glycaemic Index (GI) is a system of ranking carbohydrate rich foods based on the overall effect that they have on blood glucose levels. Foods with a low GI are absorbed slowly, producing smaller rises in blood sugar levels and helping to maintain even blood glucose levels between meals. Foods with a high GI are absorbed quickly, resulting in swifter and higher peaks of blood sugar levels, which are not desirable in people with diabetes.

Foods are given a GI number according to their effect on blood glucose levels. They are measured against a 50g glucose load e.g. 275 ml Lucozade which has a GI value of 100. The GI lists for carbohydrate foods divide them into low, medium and high GI categories. A GI of less than 55 is ranked in the low category, GI values between 56 and 69 are ranked as medium and GI values over 70 are high GI.

> It is easier just to group foods into the low, medium and high categories, and then work on adjusting your diet by trying to include more low GI foods and fewer high GI choices rather than getting too anxious about the exact values of all the different foods.

There are a number of benefits to be gained by including low GI foods in your diet.

- Carbohydrate is absorbed more slowly resulting in modest rises in blood glucose levels after meals and helping to maintain even blood glucose levels between meals. This helps to reduce the risk of hypoglycaemia between meals.
- The improved blood glucose levels may help to reduce the incidence of Type 2 diabetes in those people who are at risk.
- Low GI foods make you feel full for longer which results in eating less.
- There are benefits for weight loss among overweight people.
- People who follow low GI diets have improved levels of 'good' cholesterol and a lower incidence of heart disease.

❑ What other factors affect GI?

There are several other factors that affect the GI value of a food. Determining the GI value of a meal is not as easy as reading a number off a chart.

The overall nutrient content of a food will affect its GI. Fat and protein affect the absorption of carbohydrate and lower the overall GI value. Chocolate, which has a high sugar content, has a medium GI because of its high fat content. Potato crisps and chips, which have a high fat content, have lower GI values than low-fat jacket potatoes. Milk and dairy products have low GI values because of their protein and fat content. This doesn't mean that we should be on a daily diet of chocolate, crisps and milk! We have to consider all the Guiding Principles (see p27), not one in isolation. In other words, don't choose low GI foods, then blow all your good work with a high fat/high sugar diet.

Cooking methods, food processing, the degree of ripeness of a fruit and the variety of a vegetable or grain will all affect a food's GI rating. Canned beans have a higher GI value than dried beans that are soaked before cooking. The riper a portion of fruit is, the higher the GI value. The structure and texture of a carbohydrate have an effect on the GI rating: pasta and durum wheat have low values. Wholegrain cereals and high-fibre foods act as a barrier to slow down the absorption of carbohydrate. Mixed grain breads containing wholegrains have a lower GI value than wholemeal breads which contain ground up/milled wholegrains. Basmati rice has a lower GI than other long and short grain rices.

Try to include at least one low GI food at every meal. For people with diabetes, before, during and immediately after exercise are perfect times to go for foods with high GI values, as this is exactly when a quicker absorption of carbohydrate into the bloodstream is needed.

THE GI RATINGS FOR SOME COMMON FOODS:

Low GI

Apples, bananas, cherries, grapefruit, kiwi fruit, oranges, peaches, pears, dried apricots

Beans (including baked beans, butter beans, kidney beans), chick peas, lentils, pearl barley

Pasta made from durum wheat (fettuccine, lasagne, noodles, spaghetti)

Sweet potato

Peas, sweetcorn, boiled carrots

Porridge, oats and oat bran

Milk and low fat yoghurts

Soya 'milk' and products

Peanuts

High fibre cereals (All Bran, Sultana Bran) and Special K

Multigrain bread

Medium GI

Melon, pineapple, raisins, sultanas

Couscous

Basmati rice

Boiled and new potatoes

Plain biscuits, Ryvitas, crumpets, croissants

Muesli, wholegrain cereals (Shredded Wheat, Shreddies, Weetabix)

Pitta bread, stoneground bread, rye bread

Chapattis made with wholegrain flour

Ice cream, honey, jam, chocolate

High GI

White bread, bagels, baguette, wholemeal bread, brown bread

White and brown rices

Cornflakes, Cheerios, Coco Pops, Rice Krispies, puffed wheat

Mashed potato, baked potato, chipped potatoes

Swede, parsnip

lifestyle and exercise

by Graham Toms, Consultant Physician and Diabetologist, Newham University Hospital NHS Trust

INTRODUCTION

I have observed many people with Type 2 diabetes transform the quality of their life by making changes to their lifestyle. I have also observed people with diabetes fail to take control of their condition, and enter a cycle of progressive weight gain, poor diabetes control, deteriorating cardiovascular fitness, and increasing disability (for example heart disease and/or poor mobility). A lot of these people later regretted not having been more pro-active about their lifestyle, and wished they could 'put the clock back'. There's no reason to get to this stage.

In this section, I am going to focus upon the importance of regular physical activity and discuss how exercise should be regarded as an essential treatment for Type 2 diabetes. In addition, there is now very strong medical evidence to suggest that the development of Type 2 diabetes can be delayed or prevented by regular exercise! So this section is both for people who are at risk of developing diabetes and those who already have the condition.

WHAT IS A 'HEALTHY LIFESTYLE'?

- Healthy eating
- Regular physical activity
- Keeping your weight under control
- Avoiding smoking
- Keeping your alcohol intake to a safe limit

You probably associate 'healthy lifestyle' with a desire to feel fit and well on a day-to-day basis, and a desire to reduce the future risk of diseases that impair quality of life or are life-shortening. For Type 2 diabetes, it has now been proven beyond any doubt by major clinical research studies that both the development of the disease and its successful management are inextricably linked to lifestyle, and in particular weight management. With the epidemic of obesity and Type 2 diabetes well underway in the Western world, the proven link with over eating and lack of physical activity has never been more important to recognise.

> If you are overweight and want to do something about it, be aware that losing weight by dietary means alone, or by exercise alone, can be difficult. The best and proven way to lose weight is to combine sensible healthy eating with regular exercise. This way, you simply use up more calories through daily living than you are taking in through food and drink.

WHAT IS EXERCISE?

In practical terms we are considered to be physically fit if we can carry out daily tasks with no undue physical difficulty and fatigue, and still be able to participate in some form of physical recreational activity in the evening.

In the developed world, our lifestyles have become increasingly sedentary. The use of cars, TVs and computers

> The ability to participate in physical activity in the evening may sound no big deal to many of you reading this, hopefully because you are fit and well, but in my diabetes clinic over the years, the most common reason given for not exercising after work in the evenings is: 'I'm too tired.'

for home leisure and entertainment, and our increasingly stationary working days mean that regular exercise is less likely to form part of our daily existence and often has to be 'scheduled' into our lives.

There are three components to physical fitness:

- cardiovascular fitness
- muscle strength and fitness
- flexibility

Whereas almost all forms of exercise will lead to improvement in cardiovascular fitness and the strength and endurance of some of the main muscle groups, there may be little impact on flexibility unless a routine of specific muscle stretching is carried out after the exercise session. Many people are now adding techniques like yoga to their weekly fitness programmes.

To achieve all-round fitness, you should aim to follow a balanced programme which includes all three components.

HOW MUCH EXERCISE WILL MAKE A DIFFERENCE TO YOUR FITNESS AND HEALTH?

We know from studies around the world that a total of 120–150 minutes of moderate intensity exercise per week is sufficient to gain cardiovascular fitness and produce significant health benefits. Several large and well designed studies in the USA, China and Finland have all shown the same pattern of results: a reduction in the risk of coronary heart disease by 30–50% and a reduced risk of developing Type 2 diabetes.

At this point you may be wondering how hard you actually have to exercise during these 120-150 minutes. The good news is that moderate exercise can be achieved by brisk walking, as well as jogging, swimming and cycling. In research studies in China, even 'doing the laundry' qualified as moderate intensity exercise! (As long as it is done manually.)

Other benefits from regular exercise that are less well known:

- People who exercise regularly tend to sleep better and have a better sense of well-being compared to people who remain sedentary.
- Concentration levels tend to improve, helping work performance.
- Regular exercise can elevate mood and improve anxiety symptoms. This can be a very useful therapeutic effect for people with diabetes, who are more prone to depression and anxiety.
- Regular exercise can lead to an improved sex drive (libido).

WHAT TYPE OF EXERCISE IS BEST?

Any type of exercise is good, as long as it makes you feel reasonably short of breath, without undue discomfort. For example, if you are walking briskly or jogging, you should still be able to hold a conversation. You shouldn't be gasping for breath, as you will not be able to sustain this intensity of exercise for more than a few minutes, defeating the whole object. You are aiming for aerobic exercise, which means that your exercising body is not falling behind on oxygen supply, and your heart rate is moderately raised, but a long way short of its maximum.

You don't necessarily need to join a gym and start squeezing into Lycra to do exercise! Most stationary exercise bikes in the home soon become expensive clothes hangers. You can get your daily dose of exercise by simply walking out the front door and heading off round a chosen route, preferably in a local park. You might prefer jogging, cycling, swimming or taking up a sporting activity that you have enjoyed in the past e.g. football, netball or a racquet sport. Just remember that brisk walking is fine, and you might already be getting 30 minutes of this each day by walking to work and back, or by taking your children or grandchildren to school.

THE BENEFITS OF LIFESTYLE MANAGEMENT FOR TYPE 2 DIABETES

If you have Type 2 diabetes, you need to consider how you have developed the condition in the first place. You have inherited the genes for diabetes from one or both of your parents, and there is nothing you can do about that. However, the age at which you have developed the condition, and how well your blood glucose levels are now controlled are closely related to the way you eat, exercise and weigh relative to your height (your Body Mass Index, or BMI). The chances are that when you were diagnosed as suffering from diabetes, you were significantly overweight and were eating and drinking unhealthy amounts of sugar in your diet. You may not have been getting much in the way of regular exercise, either.

The plain fact of the matter is that getting Type 2 diabetes under control begins with sensible healthy eating, regular exercise and weight control. People who are particularly overweight at the time of diagnosis have the most to gain from losing weight. People who are leading the most sedentary lifestyles at the time of diagnosis have the most to gain from starting to do some walking. In some cases, these lifestyle measures may be all that's needed to bring blood glucose levels under control, and there may be no urgency at all to consider turning to drug treatments.

Although Type 2 diabetes is an inherited condition, the age at which you develop the disease is highly dependent on lifestyle factors such as body weight, diet and physical activity.

WHAT ARE THE BENEFITS OF EXERCISE FOR TYPE 2 DIABETES?

If you have Type 2 diabetes, there are several very important and useful benefits of exercise which will improve your health in the short and long term:

❑ **Your blood glucose control will improve**
When you exercise, there is an improvement in how your muscles take up glucose from your bloodstream, under the influence of insulin. Medically, this is called an improvement in 'insulin resistance'. If you have Type 2 diabetes, then you have been genetically programmed to develop 'insulin resistance' as the main process that has led to your diabetes.

❑ **Your risk of coronary heart disease will reduce**
Your body will start to burn up fat as well as carbohydrates. If you are significantly overweight (BMI greater than 30), you will start changing your body shape over time and, in particular, you will lose some inches from your waistline through a reduction in the excess fat contained within your abdomen. This reduction in your waistline measurement alone will reduce your risk of coronary heart disease! But we also know that regular exercise leads to significant reductions in blood pressure and blood cholesterol level.

> Blood glucose control can improve within days of starting an exercise programme and you will experience further improvements over time as long as you continue to exercise regularly.

❑ **You should find it easier to keep your weight under control, or lose weight**
Losing weight through dietary changes alone can be difficult to

achieve and even harder to sustain long term. If you are eating more healthily as well as reducing your average daily calorie intake, then adding some regular exercise into the equation may enable you to stick at losing weight longer than just a few weeks.

❑ **You may find you require less drug treatment**
If you are taking drug treatments to help control your blood glucose level, then following a healthy lifestyle will help you keep the dose of the drug under the maximum, or might avoid you needing to take more than one drug. Remember, no drug treatments for diabetes are effective for long if you ignore the importance of a healthy lifestyle.

❑ **You may find yourself in a favourable cycle of weight loss and improving health!**
If you start to lose weight through a combination of healthy eating and exercise then every kilogram lost will count in terms of improving the control of your blood glucose level. If you eventually lose 5–10 kg or more, the improvement can be equivalent to the effect of a drug to control your blood glucose level. Not only that, but the control of your blood pressure and blood cholesterol will also improve, and may also reduce the number of drugs you need to take to treat these aspects of your condition. The combination of these effects will substantially reduce your risk of suffering from coronary heart disease (CHD). You will experience an improvement in your fitness and general well-being, you will feel more motivated than ever to maintain your new healthier lifestyle.

Being diagnosed as having Type 2 diabetes does not have to be a wholly negative experience. If you take the right positive steps, it can lead to a new slimmer, fitter and happier you. Go for it!

FREQUENTLY ASKED QUESTIONS ABOUT TYPE 2 DIABETES

❑ **Can a healthy lifestyle help delay or avoid getting Type 2 diabetes?**

It certainly can! There is evidence from many studies that people with a physically active lifestyle are considerably less likely to develop Type 2 diabetes than people of the same age, sex and race who lead a sedentary lifestyle. People who are very obese, e.g. have a BMI greater than 35, have a much higher risk of developing Type 2 diabetes than their counterparts of normal weight.

If you have developed impaired glucose tolerance (IGT) then the results of recent well conducted studies in the USA and Scandinavia show that you can reduce your risk of progressing to Type 2 diabetes by 50% on follow up over two years, by regular exercise (150 minutes per week), healthy eating and weight loss.

❑ **Can Type 2 diabetes be reversed?**

If you have developed Type 2 diabetes then you clearly have the genetic susceptibility for the condition and this cannot be changed. However, it is perfectly possible to achieve normal blood glucose levels through adopting a healthy lifestyle, especially if your diabetes has been diagnosed recently, and you are substantially overweight i.e. the more overweight you are at the time you are diagnosed, the more potential you have to achieve

> The more obese you are, and the more inactive you are at the time your diabetes is diagnosed, the more you have to gain from exercise, healthy eating and weight loss. Many people weighing 120 kg and above have eventually regained normal blood glucose levels by losing large amounts of weight, as much as 30–40 kg, over time.

normal blood glucose levels through successful weight loss, in combination with healthy eating and regular exercise. You will, of course, find that your blood glucose levels start to rise if you stray from your healthy lifestyle routine on a regular basis.

The most dramatic results are seen in people who resort to surgery to reduce the size of their stomachs and treat their obesity. This is not to be casually recommended as a treatment for Type 2 diabetes, though the procedure does have its place for people whose life expectancy is poor unless they lose a lot of weight.

❑ **Can a healthy lifestyle help me delay or avoid getting Type 1 diabetes?**
Unfortunately, there is no undisputed evidence to suggest that following a healthy lifestyle will help you avoid or delay developing Type 1 diabetes. The loss of insulin secretion by the pancreas that causes Type 1 diabetes is not related to lifestyle in any way and, indeed, most people with symptoms of Type 1 diabetes are either normal in weight or have lost weight through the illness before it is diagnosed.

Once Type 1 diabetes has been diagnosed, a healthy lifestyle and in particular healthy eating habits are important to keep the blood glucose steady. Regular exercise is important to cardiovascular fitness and weight control, although active participation in sports like football, rugby and endurance events can require careful planning with respect to the timing and quantity of carbohydrate intake, and insulin dosage. It is advisable to discuss these issues beforehand with a diabetes specialist nurse or physician.

If you are a serious athlete aspiring to international standard, you need specialised advice and support from a diabetes specialist who has experience of working with athletes at the very highest level of sport, where daily intensive physical training lasting several hours is the norm. Whereas such a training programme might lead to very good blood glucose control in someone with Type 2 diabetes, it is an unfortunate fact that Type 1 diabetes and international standard sport do not mix at all well; the balancing act between diet and insulin treatment becomes harder, not easier. Having said that, we all know it is possible for athletes on insulin treatment to win Olympic Gold medals, our own Sir Steve Redgrave being the most famous example.

❑ Can I smoke?

Smoking is harmful to the health of the general population. It is associated with various forms of cancer, but the increased risk of lung cancer is the most well known. Even then, in the UK the number of people who die prematurely from lung cancer is only a fraction of the total number of people who die from other smoking related diseases, with coronary heart disease (CHD) being the main killer.

Smoking will compound the risk of CHD associated with the other risk factors, which are: diabetes, a raised blood cholesterol level, raised blood pressure, and obesity. If you have developed Type 2 diabetes, it is more than likely that you also have a raised blood pressure requiring treatment, and your blood cholesterol level is also likely to be above the ideal range. These have been inherited along with the diabetes itself. You may well be overweight (with a 'high risk' waist circumference, see p72) especially if you have only just been diagnosed as suffering from Type 2 diabetes. It would be bad enough if all these risk factors simply added up when they combine but, unfortunately, they tend to multiply each other.

In other words, if you have Type 2 diabetes it would be wise to face the harsh facts that you have a very high risk of developing CHD and, if you are a smoker, you should think very seriously about giving up smoking.

❑ Can I drink alcohol?

Alcohol can be taken in small amounts – 1–2 units per day. More than this and you will risk affecting your blood glucose level. As we know, the currently recommended limits for medically safe alcohol consumption are 14 units of alcohol per week for women and 21 units per week for men. If your average weekly intake of alcohol exceeds these limits over a period of time, then you have a significant risk of developing liver damage, especially if you have inherited a genetic susceptibility to liver disease.

Bear in mind that if you decide to consume your weekly 'allowance' of alcohol in one evening when out with your friends, you may put yourself in a very dangerous and vulnerable position. Not to mention losing control of your faculties or passing out, you may become very ill the next day from inflammation to your stomach lining (alcoholic gastritis) and dehydration. Binge drinking is not to be recommended for anyone! If you have diabetes, all of the above applies, but more so. With Type 1 diabetes, be aware that the combination of insulin treatment and alcohol can be very dangerous, as they can conspire together to bring down your blood glucose level below the normal range (hypoglycaemia). Basically, if you have more than a drink or two of alcohol, say 2–4 units, there is a risk that the alcohol starts to suppress your liver's ability to supply glucose into your bloodstream, which becomes increasingly important the longer it is since you had your last meal. So, if you normally have well controlled blood glucose levels, there is a risk of hypoglycaemia if you drink over the recommended limit.

A typical scenario would be for you to take your usual quick acting insulin dose to cover your evening meal, but the alcohol drunk with and/or after the meal works with the insulin to bring

It is a sad fact that every Accident and Emergency dept in any NHS hospital in the UK has to treat people suffering from the short term and long term effects of alcohol, on a daily basis.

your blood glucose level down below the normal range. You will hopefully recognise your usual warning symptoms of hypo-glycaemia in time to take appropriate action. However, if you fail to recognise the symptoms, and have been consuming a relatively large amount of alcohol, then you may lapse into a very dangerous and vulnerable state where you lose control of your senses through a combination of lack of glucose supply to the brain, and the effects of alcohol intoxication. You will then be very dependent on the actions of people around you, most likely your friends and colleagues. There is a real risk that people will assume you are simply 'drunk' when in fact you are suffering from hypoglycaemia and urgently need fast acting sugars to bring your blood glucose level up into the normal range. You may have lapsed into a half conscious state whereby you are unable to co-operate with anyone trying to give you a sugary drink or foodstuff. You now need urgent medical attention from a paramedic.

HOW TO REDUCE YOUR RISK OF SERIOUS HYPOGLYCAEMIA ('HYPO') ON INSULIN TREATMENT WHEN ENJOYING A NIGHT OUT

If this is the first time since starting your insulin treatment, for either Type 1 or Type 2 diabetes, that you are planning a special night out with family, friends or work colleagues, talk about it beforehand with your GP, practice nurse or diabetes specialist nurse. What follows is general guidance, but you may need more specific advice tailored to your individual situation.

- Make sure that at least one of your friends or colleagues knows about hypos, and what action to take if you show any signs of going hypoglycaemic. Obviously, the more people who know what to do, the better, just in case one or more of them succumb to the effects of alcohol themselves in the course of the evening.
- Have a proper meal before you start to drink any alcohol.

- Make sure you know what your blood glucose level is before you start drinking alcohol, and recheck periodically during the evening.
- If it turns out to be a long evening of drinking and dancing, you will need to eat again to avoid a hypo. Don't wait until you start to experience any symptoms. You may need at least a snack for every few units of alcohol you consume, especially if you are spending a lot of time on the dance floor.
- Drink plenty of water to counteract the dehydrating effect of alcohol.
- To try and avoid a possible hypo within the hours after you eventually get to bed, make sure you test your blood glucose again when you get home, and eat again if necessary.
- Be aware that you might go hypo many hours after you stop drinking alcohol. Test your blood glucose again when you wake up the following day. It might be wise for someone to wake you at a pre-arranged time to check that all is well.

SUMMARY: IMPROVING YOUR HEALTH THROUGH LIFESTYLE MODIFICATIONS

Exercise

- Choose an exercise programme which includes cardiovascular fitness; muscle strength; and flexibility.
- Total 120–150 minutes of moderate intensity exercise per week (30 mins a day at least 4 times a week).
- Use a pedometer to help yourself achieve an average of 10,000 steps per day.
- Moderate exercise can be achieved by brisk walking, jogging, swimming and cycling.
- If you are at risk of developing Type 2 diabetes, regular exercise (150 mins per week), healthy eating and weight loss will reduce your risk of progressing to the disease by 50%!

Smoking

- Stop smoking. Smoking is a major cause of coronary heart disease (CHD), which will compound the increased risk of CHD associated with Type 2 diabetes. If you are struggling to give up smoking, talk to your GP or practice nurse, who can advise you on the increasing range of treatments that are available.

Alcohol

- Stick to the guidelines: no more than 2 units per day for women and 3 units per day for men. Do not binge drink, but if you are on insulin treatment and you feel this is unavoidable on special occasions, there are precautions you can take to avoid serious hypoglycaemia.

living with diabetes –
frequently asked questions

by Anne Claydon, Diabetes Nurse Specialist,
Newham University Hospital NHS Trust

Here are some common questions I am asked on a day-to-day basis by the patients in my clinic.

WHAT LEVEL SHOULD MY BLOOD SUGAR BE?

Your doctor or diabetes specialist nurse will advise what the best blood sugar level is for you. Generally, I aim for my patients to be between 4 and 7. You may be asked to use a machine to test your blood sugars. Blood sugar testing allows you to see how your blood responds to diet, exercise and medication.

WHAT SHOULD I DO IF MY BLOOD SUGAR LEVEL BECOMES TOO LOW?

If your doctor prescribes insulin or certain tablets, you may have hypoglycaemia or a 'hypo' – in other words, your blood sugar goes below 4. When you have a hypo you may experience some of these symptoms:

- Sweating
- Hunger
- Palpitations
- Shaking
- Headache
- Paleness
- Tingling of lips
- Blurred vision

- Your family may notice you are not yourself and you may become bad tempered

If you feel any of these symptoms, make yourself a sugary drink using a tablespoon of sugar in a glass of water, or have a fizzy drink like Coca Cola or Lucozade. Do not take diet drinks. You may also use glucose tablets which you can buy from the chemist. Wait 5–10 minutes and if your sugar is still below 4 or you still feel unwell, repeat the advice above.

Once you are feeling better and your blood sugar is above 4, take something to eat to keep your blood sugar up, such as a couple of biscuits or crackers. If it's near a mealtime, have your meal.

Once your hypo is under control, ask yourself the following questions to try and find out what happened.

- Did you miss a snack?
- Did you not eat enough at your last meal?
- Have you been more active than usual?
- Did you drink alcohol without eating?
- Did you take too much insulin by mistake?

WHAT HAPPENS IF I GET THE FLU AND DON'T FEEL WELL ENOUGH TO EAT?

This is where 'sick day' rules come in. It may sound strange, but if you are unwell and you do not eat, your blood sugars usually rise. The golden rule is to always take your insulin and, if you are able, take your tablets.

Whilst you are ill, measure your blood sugars more frequently. If you have Type 1 diabetes and can't eat or drink and your blood sugars are rising, I recommend a visit to the hospital. It's safer to be checked out there rather than become very unwell at home. If you have Type 2 diabetes, you should be fine as long as you adhere to the following guidelines:

- Drink plenty of fluids
- Rest as much as you can
- If you can't eat solid foods, maintain an intake of carbohydrate by taking sweet drinks such as Coca Cola, drinking chocolate, fruit juices, ice cream or soup

CAN I DRIVE A CAR IF I HAVE DIABETES?

Yes. It is the law, however, to inform the Drivers and Vehicle Licensing Agency (DVLA) if you are taking tablets or insulin. You don't have to tell them if you are diet controlled only. If you are taking insulin your licence will be renewed every three years. At this point, your doctor will have to declare to the DVLA that your eyesight is good and you have not been having hypos.

You should also inform your insurance company every time your treatment changes or you may not be covered.

WHAT SPECIAL PRECAUTIONS SHOULD I TAKE WHILST DRIVING?

I recommend to my patients that they check their blood sugar before they drive even if they are only going a short distance. Keep Lucozade or another sweet drink and a snack in the glove compartment at all times in case you feel that your sugar level is dipping. Plan each journey and take delays into account. If you are driving a long distance, stop every couple of hours and check your sugar, eating if necessary. If you do have a hypo, stop the car at a safe spot, switch off the engine, remove the key and vacate the driver's seat.

MY AUNT HAD HER LEG AMPUTATED BECAUSE OF DIABETES. HOW CAN I PREVENT THIS HAPPENING TO ME?

As discussed in Part 1 of this book, Diabetes Uncovered, diabetes can result in nerve damage or a reduced blood supply to your feet. Everybody has heard horror stories about diabetes and amputations but to prevent problems with your feet it is important to care for them. I advise my patients to:

- Wash feet daily with soap and water.
- Dry them well, especially between the toes.
- Use moisturising cream on dry skin if necessary, but not between the toes.
- Apply surgical spirit between the toes if they are particularly moist.
- When cutting nails, use clippers but do not cut too short.
- If you find it difficult to cut your nails, ask to be referred for an assessment to your local foot department.
- Choose shoes with laces or velcro if possible and wear shoes that give your toes room so they are not crushed.
- Have your feet measured when buying new shoes and wear them in gradually to prevent cuts and blisters.
- Do not walk barefoot, even at home. Remember that glass you broke last week? You may not feel it if you stand on a splinter.
- Change socks and stockings daily. Do not wear socks that are too tight.
- Examine your feet daily.
- Do not smoke.

Go to your doctor or podiatrist if you find:

- Cuts, scratches or blisters.
- Any swelling or painful areas.
- Any change in colour.
- Any discharges from a cut in the skin.

Before putting your shoes on, always feel inside to make sure there are no stones.

I AM ON INSULIN AND WOULD LIKE TO CHANGE MY JOB. IS THERE ANYTHING I SHOULD KNOW?

The best advice I can give is to be honest with your future employers. If there is a health section in the application form tell them that you have diabetes.

Since the implementation of the Disability Discrimination Act people with diabetes who use insulin can apply for and work in a range of jobs previously barred to them. For example, the police force and the fire service. However, restrictions still exist in certain areas, such as the armed forces and train drivers as well as jobs that involve regularly driving heavy goods or passenger carrying vehicles. Some local authorities also ban people who use insulin from driving taxis.

When you change jobs you must let your line manager and immediate colleagues know that you have diabetes so that they may help you if you become unwell. There is still discrimination in the workplace, mainly due to lack of knowledge of diabetes. Diabetes is covered by the Disability Discrimination Act 1995. If you have a problem at work, contact Diabetes UK care line for advice.

I HAVE DIABETES AND WANT TO GET PREGNANT. CAN I JUST GO AHEAD?

Unfortunately not. When you have diabetes you need to plan for a pregnancy. It is essential that before you get pregnant, your blood glucose control is as good as possible, in order to reduce the twofold increased risk of major foetal malformation associated with diabetes. These malformations include spina bifida and major heart defects. It is very important if you have decided to try for a pregnancy that you consult your diabetes specialist nurse or physician to discuss the pre-pregnancy planning. Apart from discussing how to get the best possible blood glucose control, it will also be important to check any other treatments you might be on, for example for high blood pressure. You will be advised to take folic acid in a 5 mg daily dose. When you do become pregnant, you will be seen in a special antenatal clinic and your appointments will be more frequent than for somebody who does not have diabetes.

PRESCRIPTIONS ARE EXPENSIVE. HOW CAN I AFFORD TO BUY MY TABLETS, AS I AM TAKING SO MANY NOW?

Everybody on medication for diabetes is entitled to free prescriptions. Your doctor will provide you with an exemption certificate.

DO I GET FREE DENTAL CARE OR EYE TESTS?

There are no dental care concessions for people with diabetes. It is important, however, that you tell your dentist that you have diabetes. You must get regular check-ups as dental problems affect your blood sugars. (Remember, if you hate going to the dentist, your blood sugars may rise through stress!) On the other hand, people with diabetes are entitled to a free eye test.

I AM GOING ON HOLIDAY TO AMERICA: DO I HAVE TO PLAN AHEAD BECAUSE OF MY DIABETES?

Yes. Take enough insulin/medication with you to last the whole trip and keep it in your hand luggage. If you are going somewhere where vaccinations are needed, ask your practice nurse. These vaccinations may upset your blood sugar control for a short time. If you are on insulin you will need a letter from your doctor to explain why you are taking sharp needles on the plane. If you are crossing zone times, ask your doctor or diabetes nurse specialist for advice about taking your medication.

You may not have a fridge in your hotel room so purchase a cool bag to keep your insulin in. Remember that hot weather can bring about hypos, so you may have to adjust your medication if the weather is hot. There's no need to ask the airline to give you a special diet as they are usually too low in starch. Take your monitoring equipment with you on the plane. Carry snacks with you in your hand luggage. And have a good time!

weight management plan

by Diana Markham, Chief Dietitian, Newham University Hospital
NHS Trust & Graham Toms, Consultant Physician and Diabetologist,
Newham University Hospital NHS Trust

If you are at present overweight, a very important step towards improving your diabetes or reducing your chances of developing the disease is to reduce your weight and keep it under control. Read on to find out more about an easy approach to achieving this.

GETTING YOUR WEIGHT UNDER CONTROL

Let us look at some of the facts about being overweight or obese in relation to diabetes:

- Being overweight, ethnic origin, family history, women with polycystic ovary syndrome (PCOS) and increasing age are all risk factors for Type 2 diabetes.
- Obesity is a leading cause of insulin resistance – a term used to describe the condition where your body cannot properly use the insulin that it produces.
- Type 2 diabetes develops as a result of insulin resistance.
- Insulin resistance in turn leads to high blood glucose levels, hypertension (high blood pressure) and hypercholesterolaemia (high cholesterol).
- Around 80% of people diagnosed with Type 2 diabetes are overweight.

In common with the rest of the Western world, there is a serious problem in the UK of people being overweight. Currently more than half the adult population in the UK is overweight, with more than 20% classed as obese. What's more worrying is that the prevalence of obesity has doubled over the past 20 years and this increasing trend is set to continue, with at least 25% of adults being obese by 2010. Today, 10% of children in the UK are now being classed as obese. The knock-on effect is that children are being diagnosed with Type 2 diabetes and the numbers are rising substantially. No longer does Type 2 diabetes warrant its former title: 'maturity onset' diabetes.

It's lucky then that modifying our diet and getting more physically active reduces the risk of developing Type 2 diabetes by 50% or more. An obese person who loses 10% of their weight will enjoy the following health improvements:

- Better blood glucose control
- Lower blood pressure
- Lower body fat levels
- 10% fall in total cholesterol

HOW DO YOU DETERMINE WHETHER YOUR BODY WEIGHT IS CORRECT?

❏ Body Mass Index (BMI)

The usual method for assessing whether or not your weight is correct for your height is to calculate your Body Mass Index (BMI). In order to do this, your weight (in kg) is divided by height squared (in metres). This produces a number, your BMI. The ideal range of your BMI is between 18.5 and 24.9 kg/m². A BMI between 25 and 29.9 is termed overweight, between 30.0 and 39.9 is obese and greater than 40 is morbidly obese.

For convenience, a chart is normally used to quickly determine your BMI, by plotting your height against weight and then reading off the inset BMI value.

THE BODY MASS INDEX (BMI) CHART

	130	132	134	136	138	140	142	144	146	148	150	152	154	156	158	160	162	164
40	23.7	23.0	22.3	21.6	21.0	20.4	19.8	19.3	18.8	18.3	17.8	17.3	16.9	16.4	16.0	15.6	15.2	14.9
42	24.9	24.1	23.4	22.7	22.1	21.4	20.8	20.3	19.7	19.2	18.7	18.2	17.7	17.3	16.8	16.4	16.0	15.6
44	26.0	25.3	24.5	23.8	23.1	22.4	21.8	21.2	20.6	20.1	19.6	19.0	18.6	18.1	17.6	17.2	16.8	16.4
46	27.2	26.4	25.6	24.9	24.2	23.5	22.8	22.2	21.6	21.0	20.4	19.9	19.4	18.9	18.4	18.0	17.5	17.1
48	28.4	27.5	26.7	26.0	25.2	24.5	23.8	23.1	22.5	21.9	21.3	20.8	20.2	19.7	19.2	18.8	18.3	17.8
50	29.6	28.7	27.8	27.0	26.3	25.5	24.8	24.1	23.5	22.8	22.2	21.6	21.1	20.5	20.0	19.5	19.1	18.6
52	30.8	29.8	29.0	28.1	27.3	26.5	25.8	25.1	24.4	23.7	23.1	22.5	21.9	21.4	20.8	20.3	19.8	19.3
54	32.0	31.0	30.1	29.2	28.4	27.6	26.8	26.0	25.3	24.7	24.0	23.4	22.8	22.2	21.6	21.1	20.6	20.1
56	33.1	32.1	31.2	30.3	29.4	28.6	27.8	27.0	26.3	25.6	24.9	24.2	23.6	23.0	22.4	21.9	21.3	20.8
58	34.3	33.3	32.3	31.4	30.5	29.6	28.8	28.0	27.2	26.5	25.8	25.1	24.5	23.8	23.2	22.7	22.1	21.6
60	35.5	34.4	33.4	32.4	31.5	30.6	29.8	28.9	28.1	27.4	26.7	26.0	25.3	24.7	24.0	23.4	22.9	22.3
62	36.7	35.6	34.5	33.5	32.6	31.6	30.7	29.9	29.1	28.3	27.6	26.8	26.1	25.5	24.8	24.2	23.6	23.1
64	37.9	36.7	35.6	34.6	33.6	32.7	31.7	30.9	30.0	29.2	28.4	27.7	27.0	26.3	25.6	25.0	24.4	23.8
66	39.1	37.9	36.8	35.7	34.7	33.7	32.7	31.8	31.0	30.1	29.3	28.6	27.8	27.1	26.4	25.8	25.1	24.5
68	40.2	39.0	37.9	36.8	35.7	34.7	33.7	32.8	31.9	31.0	30.2	29.4	28.7	27.9	27.2	26.6	25.9	25.3
70	41.4	40.2	39.0	37.8	36.8	35.7	34.7	33.8	32.8	32.0	31.1	30.3	29.5	28.8	28.0	27.3	26.7	26.0
72	42.6	41.3	40.1	38.9	37.8	36.7	35.7	34.7	33.8	32.9	32.0	31.2	30.4	29.6	28.8	28.1	27.4	26.8
74	43.8	42.5	41.2	40.0	38.9	37.8	36.7	35.7	34.7	33.8	32.9	32.0	31.2	30.4	29.6	28.9	28.2	27.5
76	45.0	43.6	42.3	41.1	39.9	38.8	37.7	36.7	35.7	34.7	33.8	32.9	32.0	31.2	30.4	29.7	29.0	28.3
78	46.2	44.8	43.4	42.2	41.0	39.8	38.7	37.6	36.6	35.6	34.7	33.8	32.9	32.1	31.2	30.5	29.7	29.0
80	47.3	45.9	44.6	43.3	42.0	40.8	39.7	38.6	37.5	36.5	35.6	34.6	33.7	32.9	32.0	31.3	30.5	29.7
82	48.5	47.1	45.7	44.3	43.1	41.8	40.7	39.5	38.5	37.4	36.4	35.5	34.6	33.7	32.8	32.0	31.2	30.5
84	49.7	48.2	46.8	45.4	44.1	42.9	41.7	40.5	39.4	38.3	37.3	36.4	35.4	34.5	33.6	32.8	32.0	31.2
86	50.9	49.4	47.9	46.5	45.2	43.9	42.7	41.5	40.3	39.3	38.2	37.2	36.3	35.3	34.4	33.6	32.8	32.0
88	52.1	50.5	49.0	47.6	46.2	44.9	43.6	42.4	41.3	40.2	39.1	38.1	37.1	36.2	35.3	34.4	33.5	32.7
90	53.3	51.7	50.1	48.7	47.3	45.9	44.6	43.4	42.2	41.1	40.0	39.0	37.9	37.0	36.1	35.2	34.3	33.5
92	54.4	52.8	51.2	49.7	48.3	46.9	45.6	44.4	43.2	42.0	40.9	39.8	38.8	37.8	36.9	35.9	35.1	34.2
94	55.6	53.9	52.4	50.8	49.4	48.0	46.6	45.3	44.1	42.9	41.8	40.7	39.6	38.6	37.7	36.7	35.8	34.9
96	56.8	55.1	53.5	51.9	50.4	49.0	47.6	46.3	45.0	43.8	42.7	41.6	40.5	39.4	38.5	37.5	36.6	35.7
98	58.0	56.2	54.6	53.0	51.5	50.0	48.6	47.3	46.0	44.7	43.6	42.4	41.3	40.3	39.3	38.3	37.3	36.4
100	59.2	57.4	55.7	54.1	52.5	51.0	49.6	48.2	46.9	45.7	44.4	43.3	42.2	41.1	40.1	39.1	38.1	37.2
102	60.4	58.5	56.8	55.1	53.6	52.0	50.6	49.2	47.9	46.6	45.3	44.1	43.0	41.9	40.9	39.8	38.9	37.9
104	61.5	59.7	57.9	56.2	54.6	53.1	51.6	50.2	48.8	47.5	46.2	45.0	43.9	42.7	41.7	40.6	39.6	38.7
106	62.7	60.8	59.0	57.3	55.7	54.1	52.6	51.1	49.7	48.4	47.1	45.9	44.7	43.6	42.5	41.4	40.4	39.4
108	63.9	62.0	60.1	58.4	56.7	55.1	53.6	52.1	50.7	49.3	48.0	46.7	45.5	44.4	43.3	42.2	41.2	40.2
110	65.1	63.1	61.3	59.5	57.8	56.1	54.6	53.0	51.6	50.2	48.9	47.6	46.4	45.2	44.1	43.0	41.9	40.9
112	66.3	64.3	62.4	60.6	58.8	57.1	55.5	54.0	52.5	51.1	49.8	48.5	47.2	46.0	44.9	43.8	42.7	41.6
114	67.5	65.4	63.5	61.6	59.9	58.2	56.5	55.0	53.5	52.0	50.7	49.3	48.1	46.8	45.7	44.5	43.4	42.4
116	68.6	66.6	64.6	62.7	60.9	59.2	57.5	55.9	54.4	53.0	51.6	50.2	48.9	47.7	46.5	45.3	44.2	43.1
118	69.8	67.7	65.7	63.8	62.0	60.2	58.5	56.9	55.4	53.9	52.4	51.1	49.8	48.5	47.3	46.1	45.0	43.9
120	71.0	68.9	66.8	64.9	63.0	61.2	59.5	57.9	56.3	54.8	53.3	51.9	50.6	49.3	48.1	46.9	45.7	44.6
122	72.2	70.0	67.9	66.0	64.1	62.2	60.5	58.8	57.2	55.7	54.2	52.8	51.4	50.1	48.9	47.7	46.5	45.4
124	73.4	71.2	69.1	67.0	65.1	63.3	61.5	59.8	58.2	56.6	55.1	53.7	52.3	51.0	49.7	48.4	47.2	46.1
126	74.6	72.3	70.2	68.1	66.2	64.3	62.5	60.8	59.1	57.5	56.0	54.5	53.1	51.8	50.5	49.2	48.0	46.8
128	75.7	73.5	71.3	69.2	67.2	65.3	63.5	61.7	60.0	58.4	56.9	55.4	54.0	52.6	51.3	50.0	48.8	47.6
130	76.9	74.6	72.4	70.3	68.3	66.3	64.5	62.7	61.0	59.3	57.8	56.3	54.8	53.4	52.1	50.8	49.5	48.3
132	78.1	75.8	73.5	71.4	69.3	67.3	65.5	63.7	61.9	60.3	58.7	57.1	55.7	54.2	52.9	51.6	50.3	49.1
134	79.3	76.9	74.6	72.4	70.4	68.4	66.5	64.6	62.9	61.2	59.6	58.0	56.5	55.1	53.7	52.3	51.1	49.8
136	80.5	78.1	75.7	73.5	71.4	69.4	67.4	65.6	63.8	62.1	60.4	58.9	57.3	55.9	54.5	53.1	51.8	50.6
	4'3"	4'4"	4'5"	4'5½"	4'6"	4'7"	4'8"	4'9"	4'9½"	4'10"	4'11"	5'	5'1"	5'1½"	5'2"	5'3"	5'4"	5'4½'

Weight in Kgs

Height in cm

166	168	170	172	174	176	178	180	182	184	186	188	190	192	194	196	198	200	
14.5	14.2	13.8	13.5	13.2	12.9	12.6	12.3	12.1	11.8	11.6	11.3	11.1	10.9	10.6	10.4	10.2	10.0	6st 4lb
15.2	14.9	14.5	14.2	13.9	13.6	13.3	13.0	12.7	12.4	12.1	11.9	11.6	11.4	11.2	10.9	10.7	10.5	6st 8lb
16.0	15.6	15.2	14.9	14.5	14.2	13.9	13.6	13.3	13.0	12.7	12.4	12.2	11.9	11.5	11.5	11.2	11.0	6st 13lb
16.7	16.3	15.9	15.5	15.2	14.9	14.5	14.2	13.9	13.6	13.3	13.0	12.7	12.5	12.2	12.0	11.7	11.5	7st 3lb
17.4	17.0	16.6	16.2	15.9	15.5	15.1	14.8	14.5	14.2	13.9	13.6	13.3	13.0	12.8	12.5	12.2	12.0	7st 8lb
18.1	17.7	17.3	16.9	16.5	16.1	15.8	15.4	15.1	14.8	14.5	14.1	13.9	13.6	13.3	13.0	12.8	12.5	7st 12lb
18.9	18.4	18.0	17.6	17.2	16.8	16.4	16.0	15.7	15.4	15.0	14.7	14.4	14.1	13.8	13.5	13.3	13.0	8st 3lb
19.6	19.1	18.7	18.3	17.8	17.4	17.0	16.7	16.3	15.9	15.6	15.3	15.0	14.6	14.3	14.1	13.8	13.5	8st 7lb
20.3	19.8	19.4	18.9	18.5	18.1	17.7	17.3	16.9	16.5	16.2	15.8	15.5	15.2	14.9	14.6	14.3	14.0	8st 11lb
21.0	20.5	20.1	19.6	19.2	18.7	18.3	17.9	17.5	17.1	16.8	16.4	16.1	15.7	15.4	15.1	14.8	14.5	9st 2lb
21.8	21.3	20.8	20.3	19.8	19.4	18.9	18.5	18.1	17.7	17.3	17.0	16.6	16.3	15.9	15.6	15.3	15.0	9st 6lb
22.5	22.0	21.5	21.0	20.5	20.0	19.6	19.1	18.7	18.3	17.9	17.5	17.2	16.8	16.5	16.1	15.8	15.5	9st 11lb
23.2	22.7	22.1	21.6	21.1	20.7	20.2	19.8	19.3	18.9	18.5	18.1	17.7	17.4	17.0	16.7	16.3	16.0	10st 1lb
24.0	23.4	22.8	22.3	21.8	21.3	20.8	20.4	19.9	19.5	19.1	18.7	18.3	17.9	17.6	17.2	16.8	16.5	10st 6lb
24.7	24.1	23.5	23.0	22.5	22.0	21.5	21.0	20.5	20.1	19.7	19.2	18.8	18.4	18.1	17.7	17.3	17.0	10st 10lb
25.4	24.8	24.2	23.7	23.1	22.6	22.1	21.6	21.1	20.7	20.2	19.8	19.4	19.0	18.6	18.2	17.9	17.5	11st
26.1	25.5	24.9	24.3	23.8	23.2	22.7	22.2	21.7	21.3	20.8	20.4	19.9	19.5	19.1	18.7	18.4	18.0	11st 5lb
26.9	26.2	25.6	25.0	24.4	23.9	23.4	22.8	22.3	21.9	21.4	20.9	20.5	20.1	19.7	19.3	18.9	18.5	11st 9lb
27.6	26.9	26.3	25.7	25.1	24.5	24.0	23.5	22.9	22.4	22.0	21.5	21.1	20.6	20.2	19.8	19.4	19.0	12st
28.3	27.6	27.0	26.4	25.8	25.2	24.6	24.1	23.5	23.0	22.5	22.1	21.6	21.2	20.7	20.3	19.9	19.5	12st 4lb
29.0	28.3	27.7	27.0	26.4	25.8	25.2	24.7	24.2	23.6	23.1	22.6	22.2	21.7	21.3	20.8	20.4	20.0	12st 8lb
29.8	29.1	28.4	27.7	27.1	26.5	25.9	25.3	24.8	24.2	23.7	23.2	22.7	22.2	21.8	21.3	20.9	20.5	12st 13lb
30.5	29.8	29.1	28.4	27.7	27.1	26.5	25.9	25.4	24.8	24.3	23.8	23.3	22.8	22.3	21.9	21.4	21.0	13st 3lb
31.2	30.5	29.8	29.1	28.4	27.8	27.1	26.5	26.0	25.4	24.9	24.3	23.8	23.3	22.9	22.4	21.9	21.5	13st 8lb
31.9	31.2	30.4	29.7	29.1	28.4	27.8	27.2	26.6	26.0	25.4	24.9	24.4	23.9	23.4	22.9	22.4	22.0	13st 12lb
32.7	31.9	31.1	30.4	29.7	29.1	28.4	27.8	27.2	26.6	26.0	25.5	24.9	24.4	23.9	23.4	23.0	22.5	14st 2lb
33.4	32.6	31.8	31.1	30.4	29.7	29.0	28.4	27.8	27.2	26.6	26.0	25.5	25.0	24.4	23.9	23.5	23.0	14st 7lb
34.1	33.3	32.5	31.8	31.0	30.3	29.7	29.0	28.4	27.8	27.2	26.6	26.0	25.5	25.0	24.5	24.0	23.5	14st 11lb
34.8	34.0	33.2	32.4	31.7	31.0	30.3	29.6	29.0	28.4	27.7	27.2	26.6	26.0	25.5	25.0	24.5	24.0	15st 2lb
35.6	34.7	33.9	33.1	32.4	31.6	30.9	30.2	29.6	28.9	28.3	27.7	27.1	26.6	26.0	25.5	25.0	24.5	15st 6lb
36.3	35.4	34.6	33.8	33.0	32.3	31.6	30.9	30.2	29.5	28.9	28.3	27.7	27.1	26.6	26.0	25.5	25.0	15st 11lb
37.0	36.1	35.3	34.5	33.7	32.9	32.2	31.5	30.8	30.1	29.5	28.9	28.3	27.7	27.1	26.6	26.0	25.5	16st 1lb
37.7	36.8	36.0	35.2	34.4	33.6	32.8	32.1	31.4	30.7	30.1	29.4	28.8	28.2	27.6	27.1	26.5	26.0	16st 5lb
38.5	37.6	36.7	35.8	35.0	34.2	33.5	32.7	32.0	31.3	30.6	30.0	29.4	28.8	28.2	27.6	27.0	26.5	16st 10lb
39.2	38.3	37.4	36.5	35.7	34.9	34.1	33.3	32.6	31.9	31.2	30.6	29.9	29.3	28.7	28.1	27.5	27.0	17st
39.9	39.0	38.1	37.2	36.3	35.5	34.7	34.0	33.2	32.5	31.8	31.1	30.5	29.8	29.2	28.6	28.1	27.5	17st 5lb
40.6	39.7	38.8	37.9	37.0	36.2	35.3	34.6	33.8	33.1	32.4	31.7	31.0	30.4	29.8	29.2	28.6	28.0	17st 9lb
41.4	40.4	39.4	38.5	37.7	36.8	36.0	35.2	34.4	33.7	33.0	32.3	31.6	30.9	30.3	29.7	29.1	28.5	17st 13lb
42.1	41.1	40.1	39.2	38.3	37.4	36.6	35.8	35.0	34.3	33.5	32.8	32.1	31.5	30.8	30.2	29.6	29.0	18st 4lb
42.8	41.8	40.8	39.9	39.0	38.1	37.2	36.4	35.6	34.9	34.1	33.4	32.7	32.0	31.4	30.7	30.1	29.5	18st 8lb
43.5	42.5	41.5	40.6	39.6	38.7	37.9	37.0	36.2	35.4	34.7	34.0	33.2	32.6	31.9	31.2	30.6	30.0	18st 13lb
44.3	43.2	42.2	41.2	40.3	39.4	38.5	37.7	36.8	36.0	35.3	34.5	33.8	33.1	32.4	31.8	31.1	30.5	19st 3lb
45.0	43.9	42.9	41.9	41.0	40.0	39.1	38.3	37.4	36.6	35.8	35.1	34.3	33.6	32.9	32.3	31.6	31.0	19st 7lb
45.7	44.6	43.6	42.6	41.6	40.7	39.8	38.9	38.0	37.2	36.4	35.6	34.9	34.2	33.5	32.8	32.1	31.5	19st 12lb
46.5	45.4	44.3	43.3	42.3	41.3	40.4	39.5	38.6	37.8	37.0	36.2	35.5	34.7	34.0	33.3	32.6	32.0	20st 2lb
47.2	46.1	45.0	43.9	42.9	42.0	41.0	40.1	39.2	38.4	37.6	36.8	36.0	35.3	34.5	33.8	33.2	32.5	20st 7lb
47.9	46.8	45.7	44.6	43.6	42.6	41.7	40.7	39.9	39.0	38.2	37.3	36.6	35.8	35.1	34.4	33.7	33.0	20st 11lb
48.6	47.5	46.4	45.3	44.3	43.3	42.3	41.4	40.5	39.6	38.7	37.9	37.1	36.3	35.6	34.9	34.2	33.5	21st 1lb
49.4	48.2	47.1	46.0	44.9	43.9	42.9	42.0	41.1	40.2	39.3	38.5	37.7	36.9	36.1	35.4	34.7	34.0	21st 5lb

| 5'5" | 5'6" | 5'7" | 5'8" | 5'8½" | 5'9" | 5'10" | 5'11" | 6' | 6'½" | 6'1" | 6'2" | 6'3" | 6'4" | 6'4½" | 6'5" | 6'6" | 6'7" |

Height in feet and inches

(Right-side vertical category labels: Underweight · OK · Overweight · Obese)

Weight in stones and pounds

Everybody with diabetes and a BMI over 25 is at risk of cardiovascular complications.

For Asian people, the ideal range for BMI is 18.5–22.9. A BMI of 23.0–24.9 is overweight, between 25.0–34.9 is obese and greater than 35.0 is morbidly obese.

☐ **Waist circumference**

Another assessment method used to determine whether your health is at risk is your waist circumference measurement. A high waist circumference indicates the presence of abdominal fat and is a good predictor of increased risk of developing Type 2 diabetes, cardiovascular disease, high cholesterol and hypertension (high blood pressure).

Health risks are associated with the following waist circumferences:
Men greater than 94 cm (37")
Women greater than 80 cm (32")
Asian men greater than 90 cm (36")
Asian women greater than 80 cm (32")

WHAT IS THE BEST WAY FOR YOU TO LOSE WEIGHT?

Weight management involves lifestyle changes. People who are more motivated to make changes will be more successful in losing weight. You also need to set yourself achievable goals and be realistic in the changes you can make. You need to look at both dietary modifications, reducing fat, sugar and portion sizes, and increasing physical activity.

Let's consider the different scenarios.

❏ **Your BMI is in the normal range**

If your weight is within the normal BMI range then that is excellent. Keep it steady, eat healthily and make sure that you include regular physical activity.

❏ **Your BMI is in the overweight range**

If your weight is in the overweight range, then you need to look at how your weight has changed over the last 12 months. Is your weight steady at this level, or is it gradually creeping up?

If your weight is steady, then you may actually be quite happy to maintain it at this level, particularly if you have been successful in actually losing a considerable amount and are now at your 'goal' weight, even though you may be theoretically overweight. If your weight is creeping up, then you certainly need to take action to prevent further increases and ideally, reduce some of the excess.

❏ **Your BMI is in the obese range**

If you are in the obese range then you need to actively try to reduce weight. This will lead to a reduction in the health risk factors associated with obesity.

Seeking professional help and support in a weight management programme is likely to produce greater results than trying to do it on your own. You should aim to lose weight gradually e.g. 0.5–1.0 kg or 1–2 lbs per week only; 'crash' diets that result in rapid weight loss are not advisable and they aren't sustainable. You can get help from your local GP practice or via a multidisciplinary health care team involving practice nurses, diabetes specialist nurses, and dietitians. There are also a large number of private sector programme providers who can help you with weight control.

KICKSTART YOUR WEIGHT LOSS

❑ **Planning your diet**

Make realistic targets (e.g. to lose 1–2 lbs a week) and plan the way ahead so you can fit sensible eating options into your day.

- Work out your meals in advance.
- Make a list to take with you when you go shopping.
- Don't shop when you are hungry.
- Include a low GI food at each meal.
- Cook extra portions and freeze them for use another day.

❑ **Improving the daily diet of a person with diabetes**

The next step is to take a good look at the way you eat now. Let's work through an example of changing the daily diet of a person with diabetes. This person, let's call her 'Jane', has already made a number of changes to her eating pattern since diagnosis. She eats three regular meals and has a small snack in between each meal. She does not add sugar to her beverages and selects 'diet' and 'low calorie' soft drinks. She has given up the chocolate bar that she used to have mid afternoon at work, and has made an additional lifestyle change of going to the gym for 30–40 minutes two or three times a week on her way home from work. She has never smoked, and her weight is at the upper end of the normal range.

Jane's present daily meal pattern is as follows:

Breakfast:
Bowl of cornflakes with semi-skimmed milk
Low fat yoghurt
1 slice of brown toast with vegetable margarine and a little
marmalade
Cup of tea

Mid morning:
Cup of coffee
Custard cream biscuit or digestive biscuit

Lunch:
White or brown bread sandwich e.g. cheese or ham and
    tomato
Packet of crisps
Banana
Can of 'Diet' Coke
Cup of coffee

Mid afternoon:
Slice of cake or 2 biscuits e.g. bourbon or digestives
Cup of tea

Evening meal:
Grilled steak
Salad with dressing
Medium-sized portion of oven chips
Slice of apple pie and scoop of ice cream
2 glasses of wine

Before bed:
2 cream crackers and some cheese (either hard cheese or
    low fat soft cheese)
Cup of tea

You can see that there are a number of good points here.
For example:

- Regular meals
- Fruit and vegetables included
- Margarine used rather than butter
- Semi skimmed milk
- Oven chips (lower in fat than regular fried chips)
- Low sugar/sugar free soft drinks
- No sweets
- Low fat soft cheese included at bedtime snack some days

Let's see if we can improve Jane's diet further.

Breakfast:
Porridge oats served with semi skimmed milk and a portion of fruit e.g. mixed berries
1 slice of multigrain toast with olive oil spread and low sugar marmalade
Cup of tea

Mid morning:
Cup of coffee
Portion of fruit

Lunch:
Multigrain bread sandwich or a wrap with a filling of low fat cheese, chicken, or ham and salad e.g. tomato, cucumber and lettuce
or baked beans on toast
or vegetable soup and wholemeal or multigrain bread roll
'Diet' yoghurt
Portion of fruit
Mineral water
Cup of coffee

Mid afternoon:
Cup of tea
Small scone
or 2 oatcakes
or slice of malt loaf

Evening meal:
Grilled steak
Peas and grilled tomato
Small side salad with low fat dressing
Boiled new potatoes

> Fruit salad with low fat crème fraiche
> 1 glass of wine
> 1–2 glasses of water
>
> **Before bed:**
> Portion of fruit
> **or** slice of toast with low fat cheese or Marmite
> Cup of tea

What beneficial changes have been made here?

- A low GI cereal has been included at breakfast
- Brown bread has been swapped for multigrain – lower GI
- Monounsaturated margarine (olive oil based) has replaced an unspecific margarine
- Reduced sugar preserve (marmalade) chosen
- Fruit rather than biscuits mid morning
- Better lunch choices – multigrain bread, low fat fillings and more vegetables included, low fat and sugar yoghurt rather than a packet of crisps and water instead of a carbonated drink
- Mid afternoon snack has a lower GI
- Evening meal – changing the potatoes to new potatoes (low fat and lower GI), increasing the amount of vegetables and choosing a low fat salad dressing. The dessert is also lower in fat and sugar
- Alcohol quantity reduced – more water included
- Snack before bed is lower in fat.

These changes will reduce the overall energy intake of Jane's diet so she is likely to lose a little weight, too.

> Set yourself a challenge – look at your own daily eating pattern and see how you could change it for the better.

ADAPTING A RECIPE TO MAKE IT HEALTHIER

You may often be drawn to a recipe that you think looks delicious. On closer inspection, you realise that it's probably not the healthiest recipe in the world – more often than not, the fat content is too high. But don't be put off! Experiment and adapt the dish. It's actually quite simple (and fun) to come up with a mouth-watering, healthy alternative. Compare the original recipe with our adapted version and see for yourself.

❑ **The Original Recipe**

PORK CASSEROLE (serves 4)

> 4 thick belly pork strips (600 g), trimmed of skin and
>   excess fat
> 6 rashers of streaky bacon, rind removed and cut into
>   small pieces
> 1 tbsp (15 ml) oil
> 1 clove garlic
> 2 medium onions, finely chopped
> 1 large cooking apple
> 150 ml dry cider
> salt and pepper

1. Preheat the oven to 170 degrees C.
2. Heat the oil in a pan and cook the pork strips until well browned. Put aside in a large shallow casserole dish.
3. Fry the bacon and then place over the pork strips.
4. Finely chop the garlic and add to the chopped onion. Spread over the pork and bacon.
5. Peel and slice the cooking apple and layer this over the pork, bacon and onion.
6. Season with a little salt and pepper.

7. Pour over 150 ml of dry cider.
8. Put a lid on the casserole and cook in the oven for about 1 hour.

❑ **Now see how this recipe could be made healthier...**

THE HEALTHY RECIPE
(Differences highlighted in bold)

4 lean pork steaks (400 g)
4 rashers of back bacon, trimmed
1 tsp olive oil
1 clove garlic
2 medium onions, finely chopped
400g can of cannellini beans, drained
1 large cooking apple, peeled and sliced
150 ml dry cider
1 tsp mixed dried herbs
pepper

1. Preheat the oven to 170 degrees C.
2. Heat the oil in a non-stick pan and cook the pork steaks until well browned. Put aside in a large shallow casserole dish.
3. Fry the bacon **(without adding any extra oil to the pan)** and then place on the pork steaks.
4. Finely chop the garlic and add it to the onions and spread over the pork and bacon.
5. **Empty the beans over the pork and bacon mixture.**
6. Layer the apple over the other ingredients.
7. **Sprinkle the dried herbs over and freshly milled black pepper.**
8. Pour over 150 ml dry cider.
9. Place a lid on the casserole and cook in the oven for about 1 hour.

❑ **What are the differences between the two dishes?**

- *Lower fat:* The original recipe is high in fat, using belly pork as the main ingredient and streaky bacon. Although the amount of oil in the recipe is not too excessive, it could be reduced, certainly if a non-stick pan is used for cooking. By making the changes in the second recipe, the fat content has been reduced dramatically by selecting leaner cuts of meat, and a smaller quantity of meat per person. Compare the difference: the fat content of the original recipe is around 55 gram/serving, whilst the fat content of the second recipe is around 16 gram/serving.

- *Healthier fat:* The only oil used in the healthy recipe is a monounsaturated variety, olive oil, rather than the non-specified oil of the original recipe.

- *Lower salt:* The salt content of the original recipe is high as bacon is included and additional salt added to the dish. In the healthy recipe, herbs have been used for flavouring instead of salt, resulting in a much lower salt content.

- *Higher GI:* Beans have been added to the healthy recipe to compensate for the smaller meat portions. This adds protein and fibre to the dish, whilst lowering the GI value at the same time – and it adds even more flavour and texture to the finished dish.

Not that difficult, is it? Have a look at some of your own favourite recipes and see how you can adapt them to make them healthier by reducing the fat, sugar and salt content.

SUMMARY: DIABETES DIET

- Make sure that you have three meals per day – don't miss meals.
- Reduce the amount of food you eat at main meals and as snacks.
- Use a smaller plate at mealtimes.
- Reduce your portion sizes of meat, chicken and fish to a quantity that would fit into the palm of your hand. Examples are 4 oz/120 g meat or oily fish, 6 oz/175 g white fish, 2 oz hard cheese, 4 oz cottage cheese or 2 eggs.
- Fill up on larger portions of vegetables and salads – aim to cover half your plate with them. Divide the other half between carbohydrate and protein foods.
- Have something to drink with your meal; it will also help to fill you up. Drinking a glass of water before a meal also helps in this way.
- If you need a snack between meals, then go for a portion of fruit.
- Avoid high fat snacks e.g. crisps, nuts and other savoury items like chevda and samosas.
- Drink plenty of suitable fluids throughout the day.
- Reduce the amount of fat and oil that you use in food preparation and cooking.
- Select low fat products e.g. lean cuts of meat, low fat dairy products, reduced fat spreading margarines.
- Only treat yourself to sweets and desserts occasionally.

KICKSTART YOUR EXERCISE REGIME

If you currently have a sedentary lifestyle, start off slowly. Begin by walking for 10–15 minutes at a time, and gradually build up your speed, the length of time you walk, and how often. If in doubt, consult your doctor or practice nurse (especially if you have a history of heart disease) and your physical trainer if you've decided to join your local leisure facility. There may be an 'exercise on prescription' scheme available to you locally – you can be referred to such schemes by your GP, free of charge. You will be assessed by a qualified physical trainer who will then work out a programme of exercise and physical training for you, taking into account your current state of fitness and your medical conditions.

A typical gym based routine is likely to include 5 to 10 minutes each of a variety of aerobic activities e.g exercise bike, step machine and treadmill. The intensity, speed and time duration of each activity will be advised by the physical trainer and may be monitored by checking your heart rate during the activity. If you attend the sessions two or three times per week you will notice within weeks that your fitness is improving e.g you can go a little faster on the treadmill, and can manage another 5 minutes with no more effort than you experienced in week one. You may be introduced to the weight training equipment so that you can carry out some light resistance training to improve the strength of your arms, legs and trunk. This will work with the aerobic exercises to improve your all round fitness.

Don't forget that you don't need to use a gym at all to get fit! You can simply walk out of your front door wearing some sensible shoes or trainers, and start walking. There are muscle strengthening exercises you can do without equipment e.g. press ups, knee bends and trunk curls. You might wish to try out a yoga or t'ai chi class to learn how to improve your flexibility with a routine you can perform at home.

An ideal exercise programme would include a combination of the above components, tailored to your needs and preferences and incorporated into your daily living routine. The social side to exercise e.g going swimming or going to the gym may be helpful with regard to motivation and ensuring long-term success. Go for a walk or a jog with a friend of roughly similar fitness. Change elements of your exercise programme from time to time to avoid your 'routine' becoming precisely that i.e. boring! It can be motivating to have a goal to work towards e.g a local charity fun run; these are usually 2 to 3 miles in distance and you can jog as slow as you like and walk it if you wish. However, maybe you have been in your exercise programme for a few months and have decided to show yourself and the world how well you are doing, by steadily jogging the whole distance! Don't be tempted to go too fast! If you are unable to hold a conversation with the person jogging alongside you, slow down!

❑ **A few pointers**
- Decide for yourself that you really, genuinely want to make some positive changes to your fitness levels.
- Incorporate exercise into your life in practical ways, so it becomes second nature. Get off the bus or tube one or two stops earlier and walk the rest; take the stairs instead of the lift; stroll round to the corner shop on foot, not by car; banish the remote control.
- Try using a pedometer to help you achieve an average of 10,000 steps per day. You might be pleasantly surprised to find how much walking you are already doing in normal daily life. It might just inspire you to dash out for a 10 minute walk to clock up those thousand or so steps you need to reach your target.

recipes to try

3

RECIPES FOR A BALANCED DIET

Many of the recipes in this chapter have been contributed by patients and staff from Newham Univesity Hospital Trust.

When planning your meals, aim to balance the content. For main courses, have the protein food covering about a quarter of your plate and the carbohydrate and vegetables should fill the remainder of the plate in about equal quantities. If you are trying to lose weight, then alter your ratios so that the vegetables cover half the plate and the protein and carbohydrate are divided between the other half. You may also think about using a smaller size of dinner plate to help reduce the total quantities that you eat.

Don't forget about including low GI foods too – aim to have at least one low GI item at each meal.

Here are five examples of balanced meals

- Chicken curry with basmati rice and a mixed salad. Fresh fruit salad served with an option of low fat crème fraiche.

- Beef casserole with carrots, broccoli and new potatoes. Baked apple with cinnamon and reduced sugar custard sauce.

- Mixed seafood, mushroom, onion and tomato pasta (e.g. tagliatelle) served with a green salad. 'Diet' yoghurt.

- Vegetable stuffed peppers topped with grated cheese and served with pitta bread. Low sugar rice pudding.

- Multigrain bread sandwich with a filling of salad vegetables and low fat cheese, ham or chicken. 'Diet' yoghurt and an apple or banana.

starters

CHEESY CHILLI MUSHROOMS*
(serves 4)

by Sharon Harman, Receptionist, Academic Centre, Newham General Hospital
'This dish can easily be cooked on a lean mean grilling machine.
Delicious served with a grilled steak and peas.' – Sharon

> 8 large flat mushrooms
> 200 g / 7 oz low fat cheddar cheese
> 5 red chillies
> 5 green chillies

1. Preheat the grill, or grilling machine, for 10 minutes.
2. Wash and peel the mushrooms.
3. Grate the cheese.
4. Finely chop the chillies (you may wish to remove the seeds if you do not want the dish to be too hot).
5. Mix the cheese and chillies together and stuff inside each mushroom.
6. Place the mushroom flat side down on the grilling machine, or on a grill pan under a conventional grill, and cook for 10 minutes.

* Serve with pitta bread or rice as carbohydrate if you have this dish as a meal on its own rather than as a starter.

Per serving: energy 195 kcals, 15 g protein, 13 g fat, virtually nil carbohydrate

GREEK LENTIL SOUP (serves 4)

by Anna Collard, Facilitator for diabetes story telling, Newham General Hospital

'This is an easy to prepare soup – a favourite with all the family. Low fat and low GI.' – Anna

150 g / 5½ oz small brown lentils
15 ml / 1 tbsp olive oil
1 medium onion, chopped
1 large carrot, chopped
1 stick of celery, chopped
1 tsp oregano
bay leaf
salt and pepper
water
200 g can tomatoes

1. Soak the lentils for 2 hours before cooking – they will then cook more quickly.
2. Heat the oil in a large pan and fry the onion until soft.
3. Add the chopped carrot and celery.
4. Lower the heat and add the drained lentils.
5. Add the oregano, bay leaf and pepper.
6. Cover the ingredients with cold water and bring to the boil.
7. Lower the heat, place the lid on the pan, and simmer gently for 30–40 minutes until the lentils are soft and the vegetables cooked.
8. Add the tinned tomatoes, season with a little salt and cook for a further 10 minutes.
9. Serve with bread (e.g. pitta bread or French bread).

Per serving: energy 140 kcals, protein 5 g, fat 4 g, carbohydrate 22 g
Low GI

SMOKED TROUT & APPLE SALAD*
(serves 4)

> 2 red eating apples
> 30 ml / 2 tbsp French dressing
> ½ bunch of watercress
> 1 smoked trout (approximately 175 g / 6 oz in weight)
>   or 2 fillets
> fresh chives to garnish
> *for the dressing:*
> 150 ml / 5 fl oz low fat natural yoghurt
> 1 tsp lemon juice
> 2 tsp horseradish sauce
> salt and pepper

1. Wash the apples, cut into quarters and remove the cores. Slice them thinly into a bowl and toss in the French dressing to prevent them turning brown.
2. Tear the watercress into sprigs and arrange on 4 serving plates.
3. If the trout is not filleted, then remove the skin and bones. Flake the fish into largish pieces and arrange with the apple on the watercress.
4. Make the horseradish dressing by whisking all the ingredients together, and drizzle this over the trout.
5. Sprinkle the chopped chives over the top as garnish.

* Serve with bread as a carbohydrate if you have this dish as a meal on its own rather than as a starter.

> Per serving: energy 190 kcals, protein 12 g, fat 13 g, carbohydrate 7 g

WHITE BEAN & TUNA SALAD
(serves 4)

175 g / 6 oz haricot beans
sprig of thyme
bunch of spring onions
1 small carrot, cut into chunks
200 g can tuna fish
½ red onion, cut into rings
1 tbsp of chopped parsley
crisp lettuce leaves on which to serve
For the dressing:
½ tsp salt
1 clove of garlic, crushed
1 tsp mustard
2 tsp lemon juice
1 tsp wine vinegar
black pepper
15 ml / 1 tbsp olive oil

1. Put the beans in a pan and cover with a lot of water. Bring to the boil and simmer for 5 minutes. Then leave them to continue soaking for 2 hours.
2. Add the thyme, spring onions, and carrot chunks and simmer the beans for about one hour, until they are tender.
3. Make the dressing by crushing the salt and garlic together, then add the mustard, lemon juice, vinegar and pepper and then stir in the olive oil, mixing the dressing well.
4. Drain the beans and remove the onions, carrot and thyme. Put the beans in a large bowl and pour the dressing over them. Add a little salt if necessary.
5. Drain the tuna fish and break into large flakes.

6. Stir the onion rings, tuna flakes and parsley into the bean and dressing mixture.
7. Place the lettuce leaves on four plates and put the tuna and beans on top.
8. Sprinkle a little more chopped parsley on top for decoration.

Tip: This classic Italian dish can be served as a starter for a main meal or as a light lunch.

Per serving: energy 246 kcals, protein 21 g, fat 5 g, carbohydrate 23 g
Low GI

GREEK VEGETABLE SALAD (serves 4)

by Afizah Noobeebuy, Diabetes Specialist Nurse

400 g / 14 oz tomatoes, cut in wedges

½ cucumber, cut into small wedges

100 g / 3½ oz olives

200 g / 7 oz feta cheese, cut into small cubes

for the dressing:

15 ml / 1 tbsp olive oil

15 ml / 1 tbsp white wine vinegar

15 ml / 1 tbsp lemon juice

1 tbsp chopped parsley or coriander

salt and pepper

1. Combine all the dressing ingredients together in a bowl.
2. Add the tomatoes, cucumber, olives and feta cheese and toss.
3. Serve with pitta bread.

Per serving: energy 280 kcals, protein 15 g, fat 23 g, carbohydrate 3.5 g

CHICKPEA AND PUMPKIN SOUP
(serves 4)

> 1 kg / 2 lb 4 oz pumpkin
> 700 ml / 1¼ pints vegetable stock
> 1 tsp olive oil
> 1 medium onion, chopped
> ½ tsp ground cumin
> 2 tsp wholegrain mustard
> 400 g can chickpeas, drained
> shredded basil leaves to garnish

1. Preheat the oven to 200 degrees C / gas mark 6.
2. Cut the pumpkin into large wedges, leaving the skin on.
3. Place the wedges in a baking dish and bake for 40 minutes until the flesh of the pumpkin is soft and golden in colour.
4. Scrape the flesh out of the skin and place in a blender with half the stock. Blend until smooth (you may have to do this in two batches).
5. Heat the oil in a non stick saucepan over a medium heat and add the oil, onion and cumin and cook for 4 or 5 minutes until soft.
6. Add the mustard, remaining stock, pumpkin puree and simmer for 5 minutes.
7. Add the chickpeas, stir in well and cook for a further 5 minutes.
8. Serve up in individual bowls, and garnish with shredded basil leaves.

> Per serving: energy 200 kcals,
> protein 10 g, fat 4 g,
> carbohydrate 32 g
> Low GI

FIGS AND PARMA HAM* (serves 4)

40 g / 1½ oz rocket

4 fresh figs

4 slices of Parma ham

15 ml / 1 tbsp fresh orange juice

15 ml / 1 tbsp olive oil

2 tsp clear honey

½ small fresh red chilli

1. Tear the rocket into bite-sized pieces and arrange on 4 plates.
2. Cut the figs into quarters and arrange on top of the rocket.
3. Cut the Parma ham into strips and arrange over the figs and rocket.
4. Place the orange juice, oil and honey in a small screw top jar and shake until the mixture emulsifies into a thick dressing.
5. Dice the chilli having removed the seeds first. Add to the dressing.
6. Drizzle the dressing over the Parma ham, rocket and figs. Serve immediately.

Tip: You can omit the chilli if you don't want the dressing to be hot.

* Include some carbohydrate e.g. bread if you have this dish on its own rather than as a starter.

Per serving: energy: 65 kcals, protein 6 g, fat 6 g, carbohydrate 7 g

SALAD NICOISE* (serves 4)

1 small lettuce
350 g / 12 oz of tomatoes, quartered
½ cucumber, peeled and cut into chunks
115 g / 4 oz of cooked new potatoes, sliced
115 g / 4 oz cooked French beans
2 hard-boiled eggs, peeled and quartered
200 g can tuna, drained and flaked
45 g tin anchovy fillets, well drained
50 g / 1¾ oz of stoned black olives
30 ml / 2 tbsp vinaigrette dressing
1 tbsp chopped parsley

1. Arrange the lettuce leaves on four plates.
2. Then arrange the tomatoes and cucumber in layers.
3. Next add the slices of potato and French beans.
4. Place the quartered hard-boiled eggs on top and the flaked tuna fish.
5. Decorate the top of the salad with anchovy fillets and the black olives.
6. Pour over the vinaigrette dressing and garnish with chopped parsley.

Tip: This universally popular summer salad can also be served as a main course.

* Include some carbohydrate e.g. bread if you have this dish on its own rather than as a starter.

Per serving: energy 313 kcals, protein 20 g, fat 19 g, carbohydrate 8 g

CELERY SOUP* (serves 4)

350 g / 12 oz celery
15 ml / 1 tbsp olive oil
115 g/ 4 oz potatoes (peeled and cut into chunks)
600 ml / 1 pint stock (chicken or vegetable)
150 ml / 5 fl oz semi-skimmed milk
salt and black pepper

1. Remove the leaves from the celery and keep to one side. Wash the celery and chop into 2.5 cm / 1 inch pieces.
2. Heat the oil in a large pan, and add the chopped celery and potatoes. Cook for 10 minutes over a low heat with the pan covered.
3. Add the stock and salt. Cook for a further 20 minutes until the vegetables are tender.
4. Puree the soup in a blender.
5. Return to the pan, add the milk and freshly ground black pepper and bring the soup back up to the boil.
6. Before serving, add the chopped celery leaves to the soup.

* Include some carbohydrate e.g. bread if you have this dish on its own rather than as a starter to a meal.

> Per serving: energy 90 kcals, protein 2.5 g, fat 4.4 g, carbohydrate 9 g

HALEEM (serves 6)

by Indra Southgate, Clinical Nurse Specialist, Newham University Hospital NHS Trust

150 g / 5½ oz dried yellow split peas
115 g / 4 oz lentils
750 g / 1 lb 10 oz lean lamb
1 large onion, diced
2 tsp olive oil
4 tsp garam masala
4 tsp ground cumin
85 g / 3 oz oatmeal
juice of 1 lemon
1 shallot, diced
salt
coriander leaves to garnish

1. Place the split peas and lentils in a pan with plenty of water and some salt. Bring to the boil and cook for 30 minutes.
2. Cut the lamb into cubes.
3. Fry the onion in the olive oil in a wok for a few minutes and then add the lamb.
4. Cook the meat for a few minutes and add the garam masala and ground cumin.
5. When the dhal is cooked, add the lamb with 1½ litres / 2¾ pints of water, place in a pressure cooker and cook for 20 minutes at high pressure. Allow to cool before removing the pressure cooker lid.
6. Add the oats and 150 ml / 5 fl oz of water. Bring to the boil until it thickens to a nice soup.
7. Serve hot and stir in lemon juice, chopped shallot and coriander leaves. Chilli sauce may also be added.

Per serving: energy 414 kcals, protein 14 g, fat 14 g, carbohydrate 35 g
Low GI

SMOKED FISH PÂTÉ* (serves 4)

1 smoked mackerel fillet

1 smoked trout fillet

125 g / 4½ oz smoked salmon bits

juice of half a lemon

125 g / 4½ oz low fat soft cheese (e.g. low fat Philadelphia)

¼ teaspoon of nutmeg

salt and black pepper

to garnish:

watercress

wedges of lemon

1. Remove the skin from the mackerel and trout fillet.
2. Place the mackerel and trout fillet pieces in a bowl. Add the smoked salmon bits. Mash the fish together with a fork.
3. Add the lemon juice and soft cheese and continue to mash together until blended.
4. Add the nutmeg, salt and pepper.
5. Put the pâté into a terrine and chill for at least an hour until firm.
6. Serve garnished with watercress and lemon wedges and slices of warm wholemeal toast.

* Including toast with the pate will provide carbohydrate to nutritionally balance this dish.

Per serving: energy 200 kcals, protein 17 g, fat 11 g, carbohydrate trace

HUMMUS (serves 4)

400 g can chickpeas
juice of 1 lemon
90 ml / 6 tbsp tahini
15 ml / 1 tbsp olive oil
2 cloves of garlic, crushed
salt and pepper
1 tbsp chopped fresh coriander to garnish

1. Drain the chick peas, reserving 2 tbsp of the liquid.
2. Place the chick peas and a tbsp of the liquid in a food processor and blend until smooth, gradually adding the remaining liquid and lemon juice.
3. Stir in the tahini and olive oil.
4. Add the garlic, seasoning to taste and blend again.
5. Spoon the hummus into a bowl and put in the fridge to chill.
6. Before serving, garnish with some chopped coriander.

Tip: Hummus is delicious spread on warm pitta bread or toasted ciabatta bread as a summer starter, or alternatively with a green salad for a light lunch.

Per serving: energy 242 kcals,
protein 10 g, fat 5 g,
carbohydrate 24 g
Low GI

main courses: meat

IRISH STEW (serves 4)

by Jean Harrington, Health Care Assistant, Out patients department, Newham General Hospital

8 lamb cutlets from the scrag or middle neck of lamb
500 g / 1 lb 2 oz potatoes, peeled and sliced
2 medium-sized onions, thickly sliced
100 g / 3½ oz carrots, peeled and sliced
1 tsp dried thyme
375 ml / 13 fl oz pint of water
salt and pepper

1. Trim the fat off the cutlets.
2. Arrange a layer of potato slices on the bottom of a heavy-bottomed saucepan.
3. Cover with a layer of onions, carrots and then meat.
4. Sprinkle with a little salt, pepper and thyme.
5. Repeat the layering process, finishing with a layer of potatoes.
6. Pour the water into the stew and place the saucepan over a moderate heat and bring to the boil.
7. Reduce the heat, tightly cover the saucepan and simmer for 2 to 2½ hours until the lamb cutlets are tender. Shake the pan occasionally during cooking to ensure that the potatoes do not stick to the bottom of the pan.

Per serving: energy 490 kcals, protein 25 g, fat 19 g, carbohydrate 30 g
High GI

LAMB AND VEGETABLE CASSEROLE (serves 4)

by Afizah Noobeebuy, Diabetes Specialist Nurse

8 lamb chops, trimmed
15 ml / 1 tbsp olive oil
1 medium onion, finely chopped
2 cloves of garlic, crushed
2 tbsp plain flour
500 ml / 18 fl oz water
1 stock cube
2 tomatoes, chopped
1 sprig of fresh rosemary
2 tsp fresh thyme
250 g / 9 oz green beans, cut into 2.5 cm / 1 inch lengths
2 sticks of celery, cut into 2.5 cm / 1 inch lengths
250 g / 9 oz carrots, cut into 2.5 cm / 1 inch lengths
salt and pepper

1. Preheat the oven to 180 degrees C, gas mark 4.
2. Heat the oil and fry the lamb chops on both sides. Remove from the pan and put aside.
3. Add the onion and garlic to the pan. Cook until the onion is lightly browned.
4. Add the flour and stir continually until the mixture is brown.
5. Add the water and crumbled stock cube and chopped tomatoes.
6. Next add the herbs, green beans, celery and carrots, a little salt if necessary and black pepper.
7. Place the lamb chops and vegetable mix in an ovenproof dish.
8. Cook in the oven for about 1½ hours until the lamb is tender.
9. Serve with potatoes.

Per serving: energy 530 kcals, protein 36 g, fat 35 g, carbohydrate 11 g

SCOUSE (serves 4)

by Graeme Wilson, Consultant Physician, Newham University Hospital Trust

'An authentic Scouse should allow a spoon to stand straight up in the bowl! For vegetarians, simply remove the meat from the recipe ingredients – this version is termed "Blind Scouse". – Graeme

450 g / 1 lb neck of lamb, trimmed of fat and cut into cubes
225 g / 8 oz braising steak, trimmed of fat and cubed
2 medium-sized onions, diced
600 ml / 1 pint of beef stock
15 ml / 1 tbsp olive oil
600 g / 1 lb 5 oz potatoes, diced
600 g / 1 lb 5 oz carrots
1 tsp fresh thyme
salt and pepper to taste

1. Heat the oil in a heavy-based saucepan or casserole dish.
2. Seal the lamb and beef cubes quickly in the oil, turning regularly.
3. When the meat is brown, add the onions and cook for 5 minutes, stirring regularly.
4. If using a saucepan, put all the ingredients into a casserole dish and add all the other remaining ingredients except the salt.
5. Add hot water sufficient to cover the ingredients.
6. Place a lid on the casserole and cook on a low heat for about 3 hours until the meat and vegetables are soft and tender.
7. Taste and adjust the seasoning.

> Per serving: energy 590 kcals, protein 47 g, fat 24 g, carbohydrate 40 g
> High GI

LAMB SHANKS AND LENTILS

(serves 4)

by Diana Markham, Dietitian, Newham University Hospital NHS Trust
'This is an easy-to-cook and warming dish for a winter's day.' –
Diana

> 8 small or 4 large lean lamb shanks
> 2 x 400 g cans whole peeled tomatoes
> 1 medium-sized onion, chopped
> 850 ml / 1½ pints beef stock
> 375 ml / half a bottle red wine
> 1 tsp dried mixed herbs
> 200 g / 7 oz lentils e.g. du puy lentils
> salt and pepper

1. Preheat the oven to 200 degrees C, gas mark 6.
2. Place the lamb shanks, tomatoes, chopped onions, stock, wine, mixed herbs and salt and pepper in a large casserole dish. Cover with a tight-fitting lid and bake for 45 minutes.
3. Add the lentils and turn the oven down to 160 degrees C, gas mark 3 and continue to cook for a further 1¾ hours until the lamb is tender and the lentils soft.
4. Serve the lamb shanks with the juices poured over them and accompanied by mashed potatoes and seasonal vegetables.

> Per serving: energy 430 kcals,
> protein 43 g, fat 9.5 g,
> carbohydrate 12 g
> Low GI.

BEEF IN A CREAM SAUCE (serves 4)

by Monette Caadan

> 500 g / 1 lb 2 oz beef (sliced into thin strips approximately
> ½ cm / ¼ inch wide)
> juice of 1 lemon
> 30 ml / 2 tbsp soy sauce
> 15 ml / 1 tbsp olive oil
> 1 medium onion, finely chopped
> 3 tbsp flour
> 400 ml / 14 fl oz of water
> 50 ml / 2 fl oz evaporated milk
> 100 ml / 3½ fl oz beef broth

1. Marinate the beef with the lemon juice and soy sauce for
   30 minutes.
2. Heat the oil in a pan and fry the marinated beef until brown.
3. Add the onion.
4. Sprinkle the flour over the beef and cook for 2 minutes,
   stirring continually.
5. Add the water and remainder of the marinating liquid.
6. Simmer until the beef is tender.
7. Add the milk and beef broth and simmer for a further
   2 minutes.
8. Serve with poatoes and vegetables.

Per serving: energy 370 kcals,
protein 37 g, fat 16 g,
carbohydrate 14 g

CHILLI CON CARNE (serves 4)

by Sharon Devlin, Library Assistant, Newham University Hospital NHS Trust
'This recipe uses some tinned ingredients which makes it quick to prepare.' – Sharon

450 g / 1 lb lean mince beef
1 Oxo cube
1 medium onion, chopped
400 g can chopped tomatoes
12 button mushrooms, sliced
150 g / 5½ oz carrots, peeled and sliced
2 tsp chilli powder
30 ml / 2 tbsp tomato puree
1 tsp garlic puree
400 g can red kidney beans, washed and drained

1. Dry fry the mince in a non-stick pan.
2. Add the Oxo cube and chopped onion and continue to cook for 5 minutes.
3. Add the tomatoes, mushrooms, carrots and kidney beans and stir well.
4. Next add chilli powder, tomato puree and garlic puree.
5. Cover the pan and simmer for 10 minutes.
6. Serve with rice.

Per serving: energy 400 kcals,
protein 30 g, fat 14 g,
carbohydrate 29 g
Low GI

PORK CHOPS IN ORANGE SAUCE (serves 4)

by Beryl Garrud, patient with diabetes

4 pork chops, trimmed

2 tsp dried sage

salt and black pepper

15 ml / 1 tbsp olive oil

1 clove of garlic, chopped

2 tsp of cornflour

250 ml / 9 fl oz chicken stock

90 ml / 6 tbsp orange juice

2 oranges, peeled and segmented

watercress to garnish

1. Season the chops with salt and pepper and sprinkle sage over each one.
2. Heat the oil in a pan and fry the garlic for a minute and then add the chops and brown them on both sides. Remove from the pan and put to one side.
3. Stir the cornflour into the pan and cook for a few minutes.
4. Gradually add the stock and orange juice and bring to the boil.
5. Return the chops to the pan, reduce the heat and add the segments from one orange.
6. Cover and cook for 40 minutes.
7. Garnish with the segments of the second orange and watercress.
8. Serve with rice and fresh vegetables of your choice.

Per serving: energy 350 kcals, protein 28 g, fat 27 g, carbohydrate 6 g

BOEUF A L'ORANGE (serves 4)

by Beryl Garrud, patient with diabetes

500 g / 1 lb 2 oz braising steak
15 ml / 1 tbsp olive oil
225 g / 8 oz button onions
115 g / 4 oz mushrooms, sliced
clove of garlic, crushed
2 tbsp flour
250 ml / 9 fl oz beef stock

for the sauce:
2 oranges
1 tbsp tomato puree
45 ml / 3 tbsp brandy
15 ml / 1 tbsp black treacle
salt and pepper
parsley to garnish

1. Preheat the oven to 160 degrees C or gas mark 3.
2. Heat the oil in a pan and fry the meat until sealed. Transfer into an ovenproof casserole.
3. Fry the onions and garlic in the same fat until golden brown, and then add to the casserole.
4. Stir the flour into the fat, cook for 1 minute and then add the stock gradually, stirring until it reaches boiling point.
5. Pare the rind from one orange, and cut into julienne strips. Cut the orange in half and squeeze out the juice. Add the rind and juice to the sauce.
6. Add the tomato puree, brandy and black treacle. Season with a little salt and black pepper. Pour over the beef and onions in the casserole dish. Place the lid on the casserole and cook in the oven for about 1½ hours.
7. Add the mushrooms – and extra stock if needed – and return to the oven for a further 30 minutes or until the meat is tender.
8. Cut the second orange into wedges and use this, and some parsley, to garnish the casserole before serving.
9. Serve with poatoes and vegetables.

Per serving: energy 340 kcals, protein 25 g, fat 18 g, carbohydrate 8 g

CARBONADE OF BEEF (serves 4)

500 g / 1 lb 2 oz braising beef, cut into 2.5 cm / 1 inch cubes
15 ml / 1 tbsp olive oil
225 g / 8 oz onions, diced
15 ml / 1 tbsp plain flour
330 ml / small can of Guinness
1 clove of garlic, crushed
1 bay leaf
8 button mushrooms, sliced (optional)
salt and pepper

1. Preheat the oven to 140 degrees C, gas mark 1.
2. Heat the oil in a large flameproof casserole dish and then add the meat, a few pieces at a time. Sear until brown, and then put onto a separate plate.
3. Add the onions and cook until brown.
4. Lower the heat and return the meat to the casserole. Stir in the flour.
5. Add the Guinness, bay leaf, garlic, sliced mushrooms (if being used), salt and pepper. Bring to simmering point, place the lid on the casserole, transfer to the oven and cook for 3 hours.
6. Mashed potatoes and red cabbage accompany this dish very nicely.

Per serving: energy 300 kcals, protein 41 g, fat 10 g, carbohydrate 7 g

SHEPHERD'S PIE (serves 4)

15 ml / 1 tbsp olive oil
2 medium-sized onions, chopped
1 medium carrot, diced
450 g / 1 lb lean minced lamb
salt and black pepper
½ tsp dried mixed herbs
15 ml / 1 tbsp chopped parsley
15 ml / 1 tbsp plain flour
15 ml / 1 tbsp tomato puree
275 ml / 9½ fl oz beef or vegetable stock
for the topping:
500 g / 1 lb 2 oz potatoes
50 ml / 2 fl oz semi-skimmed milk
25 g / 1 oz butter
25 g / 1 oz grated Cheddar cheese

1. Preheat the oven to 200 degrees C / gas mark 6.
2. Heat the oil in a pan and add the onions and carrot and cook for 5 minutes until they are soft. Add the mince and cook for a further 20 minutes until browned. Season with salt and pepper, add the mixed herbs and chopped parsley.
3. Stir in the flour, mix the tomato puree with the hot stock and add to the meat mixture and bring to simmering point.
4. Peel the potatoes and chop into chunks. Boil until soft.
5. Cream the potatoes with the milk and butter and season with salt and pepper.
6. Put the meat mixture in a lightly oiled baking dish and spread the creamed potato over the top. Sprinkle with cheese.
7. Bake in the oven for 25 minutes until the top is golden.

Per serving: energy 406 kcals, protein 28 g, fat 21 g, carbohydrate 31 g
High GI

SPICY SAUSAGE AND CHICK PEA HOTPOT (serves 4)

700 g / 1 lb 9 oz peeled potatoes
450 g / 1 lb of Frankfurter sausages
400 g can chopped tomatoes
400 g can chick peas, drained
200 g can butter beans, drained
125 g / 4½ oz sweetcorn
1 tsp Worcestershire Sauce
2 tsp dried oregano
30 ml / 2 tbsp tomato puree
25 g / 1 oz butter
salt and pepper

1. Preheat the oven to 190 degree C, gas mark 5.
2. Boil the potatoes until just tender.
3. Cook the Frankfurters following the instructions on the packet and then slice into chunks.
4. Mix the sausages with all the other ingredients except the potatoes and butter.
5. Place the mixture in an ovenproof dish.
6. Drain and slice the potatoes. Arrange the slices of potato neatly over the sausage and vegetable mixture.
7. Dot with the butter and bake for 20–25 minutes until golden brown.
8. Serve with a green salad.

Tip: This dish could also be prepared using grilled, reduced fat ordinary sausages.

Per serving: energy 700 kcals, protein 30 g, fat 37 g, carbohydrate 76 g
Medium GI

LAMB KEBABS (serves 4)

by Afizah Noobeebuy, Diabetes Specialist Nurse

500 g / 1 lb 2 oz lean minced lamb
1 medium onion, chopped
2 cloves garlic, crushed
2.5 cm / 1 inch root ginger, finely chopped
1 small green chilli, finely chopped (optional)
125 g / 4 oz natural yoghurt
salt and pepper
1 tsp cumin
8 button mushrooms
8 cherry tomatoes
15 ml / 1 tbsp olive oil

1. Mix the lamb with all the ingredients except the mushrooms, tomatoes and oil.
2. Season with salt and pepper.
3. Divide the mixture into 16 equal portions and shape into small balls.
4. Thread the lamb balls onto the 4 oiled skewers, alternating them with the mushrooms and cherry tomatoes. Brush with oil.
5. Place the skewers on a tray beneath a pre-heated grill.
6. Cook for about 12 minutes, turning regularly. Brush with a little additional oil if necessary.
7. Serve with pitta bread and salad.

Per serving: energy 260 kcals, protein 28 g, fat 17 g, carbohydrate 3 g

BEEF ROJAN JOSH (serves 4)

by Leila Badvie, Dietitian

4 cloves garlic
2.5 cm / 1 inch root ginger
15 ml / 1 tbsp olive oil
6 cardamom pods
1 bay leaf
2.5 cm / 1 inch cinnamon stick
500 g / 1 lb 2 oz lean stewing beef cut into 2.5 cm / 1 inch cubes
2 medium onions, chopped
2 tsp cumin
2 tsp ground coriander
15 ml / 1 tbsp sweet paprika
½ tsp cayenne pepper
2 tsp tomato puree
1 tsp salt
200 ml / ⅓ pint water

1. Put the garlic and ginger in a food processor with 120 ml / 4 fl oz of water and blend to a paste.
2. Put the oil in a large non-stick pan over a medium heat. Add the cardamom pods, bay leaf and cinnamon.
3. Add the beef pieces and brown on all sides and then remove and put on one side.
4. Add the onions to the oil left in the pan. Cook until brown.
5. Add the garlic and ginger paste and stir, then add the cumin, coriander, paprika and cayenne pepper and tomato puree.
6. Add the meat to the pan plus the salt and water. Stir and bring to the boil. Turn the heat down and simmer on a low heat for about 1½ hours until the meat is tender.
7. Serve with rice or nan bread.

Per serving: energy 300 kcals, protein 26 g, fat 16 g, carbohydrate 4 g

STEW PEAS AND RICE (serves 4)

by Yasmin, Stratford Ward, Newham General Hospital

'This Jamaican dish has been modified to make it healthier by not frying the meat. Traditionally spinners (small white flour dumplings) are included with this meal – omitting them makes the dish healthier.' – Yasmin

150 g / 5½ oz pig's tail or oxtail
125 g / 4½ oz of salt beef
500 g / 1 lb 2 oz shin of beef
250 g / 9 oz dried kidney beans
sprig of thyme
1 clove garlic
1 spring onion
1 chilli pepper (optional)
black pepper

1. Soak the pig or oxtail and salt beef in cold water for an hour.
2. Clean the kidney beans and wash in cold water.
3. Cut the shin of beef into cubes.
4. Put the beans into a large pan and add the soaked salt beef and pig or oxtail and the shin of beef. Add enough water to cover the ingredients completely.
5. Bring to the boil and then lower the heat and simmer until the meat is tender and the beans soft (around 3 hours).
6. Add extra water during the cooking if necessary.
7. When the meat and beans are tender, add the thyme, garlic, spring onion, chilli pepper (if included) and black pepper. There should not be any need to add salt, but taste and see.
8. Serve with rice.

Per serving: energy 310 kcals, protein 10 g, fat 24 g, carbohydrate 13 g
Low GI

MEAT BIRYANI (BEEF OR LAMB)

(serves 4) *by Iftikhar Ahmed, Senior Staff Nurse, ESSU*

1 medium-sized onion, sliced

15 ml / 1 tbsp olive oil

200 g / 7 oz lean beef or lamb, cubed

2.5 cm / 1 inch root ginger, chopped

2 medium-sized potatoes, peeled and quartered

2 cloves garlic, sliced

2 medium-sized tomatoes, chopped

1 tsp salt

125 g / 4 oz low fat plain yoghurt

1 red chilli, chopped

¼ tsp turmeric powder

½ tsp cinnamon

½ tsp cumin

1 bay leaf

4 cloves

4 black peppercorns

200 g / 7 oz basmati rice

1. Fry the onion in 1 tsp of olive oil until golden brown.
2. Add the meat, ginger, potatoes and garlic and continue frying for 2 minutes.
3. Add the tomatoes and salt and cook for a further 5 minutes until the tomatoes are soft.
4. Add the yoghurt, red chilli, turmeric, cinnamon, cumin, bay leaf, cloves and peppercorns and continue cooking for 15 minutes. (Add 150 ml / one cup of water to the mixture.)
5. Boil the rice separately until it is half cooked.
6. In a large saucepan or casserole dish spread the remaining 2 tsp oil over the base and sides. Alternate layers of rice and the meat mixture.
7. Place the lid on the saucepan/casserole and continue cooking over a low heat until the rice is fully cooked.

8. Mix well before serving.
9. Serve with a salad and raita.

> Per serving: energy 340 kcals,
> protein 10 g, fat 8 g,
> carbohydrate 34 g
> Medium GI

OXTAIL AND BEANS (serves 4)

by Yasmin, Stratford Ward, Newham General Hospital

'By boiling the oxtail instead of frying it in a lot of oil, this dish is healthier than the traditional recipe. It is still full of flavour.' – Yasmin

900 g / 2 lb oxtail
2 tomatoes
2 medium-sized onions, chopped
1 clove garlic, crushed
1 sprig thyme
1 chilli pepper
250 g / 9 oz cooked broad beans
salt and pepper

1. Boil the pieces of oxtail in 700 ml / 1¼ pints of water until tender. Add more water if necessary.
2. Reduce the sauce to a thick gravy by increasing the heat.
3. Add the tomatoes, onions, garlic, thyme, chilli pepper, salt and black pepper to taste. Stir.
4. Add the broad beans and additional water if necessary, lower the heat and cover the pan and simmer for 5 to 10 minutes.
5. Serve with rice and vegetables.

> Per serving: energy 180 kcals,
> protein 5 g, fat 8 g,
> carbohydrate 8 g

PORK ASADO
(SWEET PORK STEW) [serves 4]

by Rowena Martinez, Staff Nurse, Plashet Ward, Newham General Hospital

500 g / 1 lb 2 oz lean pork or 4 lean pork steaks
50 ml / 2 fl oz barbecue marinade sauce
30 ml / 2 tbsp rum
25 g / 1 oz sugar
2 bay leaves
1 tbsp cornflour
200 ml / ⅓ pint of water

1. Place the pork, water, barbecue marinade, rum, sugar and bay leaves in a pan and bring to the boil over a medium heat.
2. Lower the heat, cover the pan and simmer until the pork is tender – approximately 40 minutes for pork steaks, longer for a single large piece of meat.
3. Remove the meat from the pan and if you are using a large piece of pork slice it thinly. If using individual pork steaks, leave them as they are.
4. Thicken the sauce with the cornflour made into a paste with some water. Over a low heat, stir the paste into the sauce and continue to cook until the sauce has thickened .
5. Pour the sauce over the meat and serve.
6. Serve with rice and vegetables.

Per serving: energy 350 kcals, protein 25 g, fat 9 g, carbohydrate 12 g

main courses: chicken

CHICKEN WITH VEGETABLES

(serves 4) *by Harpreet Kaur, Bilingual Health Advocate*

'This is a quick dish to cook and is low in fat.' – Harpreet

> 4 chicken breasts (approx 500 g / 1 lb 2 oz), cut into 2.5 cm
>   (1 inch) strips
> 15 ml / 1 tbsp lemon juice
> 30 ml / 2 tbsp tandoori mix
> 200 ml / 7 fl oz low fat natural yoghurt
> 15 ml / 1 tbsp olive oil
> 1 red pepper, seeded and diced
> 1 green pepper, seeded and diced
> 100 g / 3½ oz French beans, chopped
> 1 tbsp fresh coriander, chopped, to garnish

1. Mix together the lemon juice, tandoori mix, yoghurt, oil and chicken.
2. Leave to marinate for 2–3 hours.
3. Put into a non-stick pan and cook on a low heat for 5 minutes.
4. Add the beans and cook for a further 5 minutes.
5. Add the peppers and cook until the chicken is cooked through.
6. Garnish with coriander. Serve with boiled rice or naan and vegetables.

> Per serving: energy 210 kcals, protein 30 g, fat 8.5 g, carbohydrate 3 g

BURRITOS WITH CHICKEN AND RICE (serves 4)

by Victoria Smart, D grade Staff Nurse in the Accident and Emergency Department, Newham General Hospital

100 g / 3½ oz rice
1 medium onion, chopped
15 ml / 1 tbsp olive oil
400 g can chopped tomatoes
2 skinless chicken breasts
100 g / 3½ oz reduced fat grated cheese
8 fresh wheat tortillas

1. Bring a pan of salted water to the boil. Add the rice and cook for 8 minutes. Drain the rice, rinse in fresh water and drain again.
2. Heat the oil in a large pan. Add the onion, rice and tomatoes and cook over a low heat until the tomato juice is absorbed.
3. Put the chicken breasts in a large pan and pour over sufficient water to cover and bring to the boil. Lower the heat and simmer for 10 minutes or until the chicken is cooked through. Remove the chicken from the pan and put it on a plate to cool a little.
4. Shred the chicken by pulling the flesh apart with two forks and then add the chicken to the rice mixture.
5. Warm the tortillas by wrapping them in foil and place on a plate over boiling water for 5 minutes or heat in a microwave for 1 minute on full power.
6. Add an eighth of the grated cheese to each of the tortillas along with the chicken and rice mixture and fold both sides in. Fold the bottom up and put a cocktail stick into the tortilla to hold it in place.

Per serving: energy 350 kcals, protein 28 g, fat 15 g, carbohydrate 57 g

COQ AU VIN (serves 4)

8 chicken thighs, skin removed
1 tbsp plain flour
15 ml / 1 tbsp olive oil
125 g / 4½ oz back bacon, trimmed and diced
8 button onions
1 clove garlic
1 sprig of thyme
1 bay leaf
375 ml / half a bottle of red wine
salt and pepper
12 button mushrooms
chopped parsley to garnish

1. Coat the chicken thighs with the flour.
2. Heat the oil in a large pan and fry the chicken thighs until browned. When cooked, place them in the bottom of a flameproof casserole dish in a single layer.
3. Fry the bacon in the pan that the chicken was cooked in and then add them to the chicken.
4. Brown the onions in the pan juices and then add these to the chicken and bacon, then add the garlic, thyme, bay leaf, salt and pepper to the chicken and pour the wine over the whole lot. Place the lid on the casserole.
5. Cook over a low heat for 45 minutes.
6. 15 minutes before the end of cooking, add the mushrooms to the casserole. If there is too large a quantity of juices in the casserole, then leave the lid off for the final 10 to 15 minutes of cooking to reduce the volume.
7. Serve the chicken garnished with chopped parsley.
8. Serve with potatoes and vegetables.

Per serving: energy 420 kcals, protein 31 g, fat 23 g, carbohydrate 3 g

CREAMY CHICKEN PASTA (serves 4)

by Deborah Sawkins, Sister on Emergency Short Stay Unit, Newham University Hospital NHS Trust

'This is a reduced fat version of a creamy pasta dish and also contains a lot of vegetables.' – Deborah

250 g / 9 oz dried penne
15 ml / 1 tbsp olive oil
2 chicken breasts, cut into small cubes
1 medium-sized head of broccoli
1 red pepper, sliced
16 button mushrooms, halved
1 tub (200 g) reduced fat crème fraiche
30 ml / 2 tbsp sun dried tomato paste
medium-sized basil leaves to garnish
Parmesan cheese to sprinkle on before serving
salt and pepper

1. Cook the penne according to the instructions on the packet.
2. Heat the oil in a pan and add the chicken and cook until browned.
3. Add the broccoli florets, sliced pepper and mushrooms and cook for 2 minutes.
4. Once the chicken and vegetable mixture is cooked through, combine it with the drained pasta.
5. Stir in the crème fraiche and tomato paste and stir well. Season with salt and pepper.
6. Garnish with the torn basil leaves and sprinkle on some Parmesan cheese to taste.

Per serving: energy 440 kcals, protein 27 g, fat 13 g, carbohydrate 56 g
Low GI

CHICKEN KORMA (serves 4)

by Iftikhar Ahmed, Senior Staff Nurse, ESSU

' The variety of ingredients in this dish means that it is a good source of protein and vitamins.' – Iftikhar

1 large onion, finely sliced

15 ml / 1 tbsp olive oil

4 chicken breasts (500 g / 1 lb 2 oz), diced.

25 g / 1 oz ginger, chopped

1 clove of garlic

1 tsp salt

2 medium-sized tomatoes

1 tsp red chilli powder

¼ tsp turmeric powder

½ tsp ground cinnamon

6 whole black peppercorns

4 cloves

¼ tsp cumin

400 g / 14 oz low fat plain yoghurt

1. Fry the onion in the olive oil until golden and then remove from the pan.
2. Add the chicken pieces, ginger and garlic and cook until browned.
3. Add the salt, tomatoes, red chilli, turmeric, cinnamon, peppercorns, cloves and cumin.
4. Cook for a further 10 minutes.
5. Mix the cooked onion in with the yoghurt.
6. Add the onion and yoghurt mixture to the chicken and cook for 5 minutes over a low heat.
7. Cover the saucepan and continue cooking for a further 5 minutes.
8. Serve with rice or nan bread.

Per serving: energy 215 kcals, protein 30 g , fat 8 g, carbohydrate 5 g

CORIANDER CHICKEN (serves 4)

by Hugh Steward, Director of Patient Support & Environment, Newham University Hospital NHS Trust

'This dish makes a super summer meal; it uses fresh ingredients, is low in fat and has powerful flavours – and it is quick to prepare.'
– Hugh

2 cloves of garlic, crushed
bunch of coriander
juice of one lime
4 chicken breasts
15 ml / 1 tbsp olive oil
for the garnish:
second lime for garnish
75 g / 3 oz (half a small pot) low fat natural yoghurt

1. In a bowl place the crushed cloves of garlic, chop most of the coriander (retain 4 sprigs for garnish), add a little salt, pepper and the juice of the lime.
2. Cut the chicken breasts into cubes, and add the infusion in the bowl.
3. Heat the oil in a non-stick frying pan or wok and cook the chicken until light brown (about 10 minutes).
4. Serve with a dessert spoon of low fat yoghurt spooned over the chicken and decorate with a sprig of coriander and a slice of lime.
5. Boiled rice and a salad or stir fry vegetables goes well with this dish.

Per serving: energy 190 kcals, protein 29 g, fat 8 g, carbohydrate 1 g

THAI CHICKEN (serves 4)

by Beryl Garrud, patient with diabetes

1 tsp cumin seeds

1 tsp coriander seeds

15 ml / 1 tbsp olive oil

4 chicken breasts

1 medium-sized onion, chopped

1 clove garlic, crushed

2 chillies, seeds removed and chopped

1 tsp paprika

15 ml / 1 tbsp Thai fish sauce

15 ml / 1 tbsp light soy sauce

1 chicken stock cube made up with 150 ml / ¼ pint water

1 can of coconut milk

1 lime, juice and zest

coriander to garnish

1. Dry roast the cumin and coriander seeds and then grind together with a pestle and mortar.
2. Heat half the oil in a pan and add the chicken. Cook until sealed, and set aside.
3. Add the remainder of the oil and fry the onion, garlic, chillies, the cumin and coriander seeds and the paprika.
4. Add the fish sauce, soy sauce, chicken stock, coconut milk and then the zest and juice of the lime.
5. Replace the chicken in the pan and simmer for about 30 minutes.
6. Garnish with coriander leaves and serve with rice and vegetables.

Tip: The energy and fat content of this dish can be lowered by using a reduced fat coconut milk rather than the standard variety.

Per serving: energy 300 kcals, protein 30 g, fat 31 g, carbohydrate 5 g

CHICKEN LEGS COOKED WITH CORIANDER AND SULTANAS

(serves 4)

by Dr Shanti Vijayaraghavan, Consultant Physician, Newham University Hospital NHS Trust

15 ml / 1 tbsp olive oil

5 cm / 2 inch cinnamon stick

10 cloves

6 whole cardamom pods

1 large onion, finely sliced

4 chicken legs or 8 thighs

1 tsp ground cumin seeds

1 tsp ground coriander seeds

150 ml / 5 fl oz tub low fat plain yoghurt

2 tbsp sultanas

salt

coriander leaves to garnish

1. Heat the oil in a large non-stick pan and add the cinnamon stick, cloves and cardamom. Stir and then add the finely sliced onion and cook until browned.
2. Add the chicken pieces and brown.
3. Add all the remaining ingredients and bring to the boil.
4. Turn the heat down low, cover and simmer gently for 20 minutes.
5. Remove the lid and turn up the heat so that the sauce is reduced in quantity and is thick in texture.
6. Serve garnished with the fresh coriander leaves and accompanied by rice and vegetables.

Per serving: energy 260 kcals, protein 30 g, fat 11 g, carbohydrate 8 g

CHICKEN IN THE POT (serves 4)

15 ml / 1 tbsp olive oil

1 clove of garlic, crushed

2 small onions, sliced

1 whole chicken (approx 1 kg/ 2¼ lb)

200 g / 7 oz carrots, peeled and cut into chunks

115 g / 4 oz small turnips, cut into chunks

150 g / 5½ oz swede, peeled and cut into chunks

150 g / 5½ oz celery, cut into 2.5 cm / 1 inch pieces

200 ml / ⅓ pint of chicken stock

375 ml / ½ bottle of dry white wine

2 sprigs of thyme or 1 tsp of dried thyme

2 bay leaves

salt and pepper

12 button mushrooms

1. Preheat the oven to 200 degrees C, gas mark 6.
2. Heat half the oil in a flameproof casserole and fry the garlic and onion until lightly browned. Remove and put to one side.
3. Add the remaining oil to the casserole and then fry the chicken whole. Turn it over so that the chicken is evenly browned.
4. Keep the chicken in the centre of the casserole and place the onions and all the other vegetables except the mushrooms around the side of the chicken.
5. Add the chicken stock, wine, herbs, salt and pepper.
6. Place the lid on the casserole and place it in the centre of the oven and cook for an hour.
7. Add the mushrooms and cook for a further 30 minutes.
8. Remove from the oven, carve up the chicken and serve with the vegetables from the pot, and some boiled new potatoes.

Per serving: energy 365 kcals, protein 40 g, fat 12.5 g, carbohydrate 8 g.

MALAYSIAN CHICKEN AND RICE

(serves 4)

by Vimi Gisby, CNS Stoma Care, Newham University Hospital NHS Trust

4 chicken quarters

2 tsp sesame oil

200 g / 7 oz rice

15 ml / 1 tbsp soy sauce

12 fresh red chillies

½ small white cabbage, cut into 5 cm / 2 inch squares

2.5 cm / 1 inch piece root ginger

3 cloves garlic, finely chopped

1 cucumber, sliced

bunch of spring onions

1. Remove the skin from the chicken portions. Place in a pan covered with water and boil for 30 minutes.
2. Remove the chicken, retaining the liquids, and rub in some of the sesame oil. Place to one side.
3. Wash the rice and place in a pan with the stock that the chicken was cooked in. Cook the rice.
4. Grind the soy sauce and remaining sesame oil with the garlic, ginger and chillies to form a paste.
5. Add the cabbage and seasoning paste to the rice and soup mixture and cook until the cabbage is still a little crunchy.
6. Slice the chicken into thin strips and decorate with spring onions.
7. Cut the cucumber into chunks.
8. Serve the chicken with a bowl of rice soup and cucumber chunks.

Per serving: energy 425 kcals,
protein 33 g, fat 10 g,
carbohydrate 50 g
High GI

BAKED LEMON CHICKEN (serves 4)

by Lyn Pratley, Diabetes Specialist Nurse

'This is a low fat dish using fresh ingredients.' – Lyn

> **4 skinless chicken breasts**
> **fresh coriander**
> **1 clove of garlic**
> **juice of 1 lemon**
> **black pepper**

1. Preheat the oven to 180 degrees C, gas mark 4.
2. Chop the coriander and crush the garlic.
3. Mix together the coriander, garlic and lemon juice and add black pepper to taste.
4. Place the chicken breasts on a large piece of aluminium foil.
5. Pour the mixture over the chicken and wrap the foil loosely around the chicken.
6. Cook for 1–1¼ hours until the chicken is thoroughly cooked.
7. Serve with new potatoes and a green salad.

> Per serving: energy 150 kcals,
> protein 28 g, fat 4 g,
> carbohydrate 0.5 g

BAKED CARIBBEAN CHICKEN WITH SPICY GRAVY (serves 4)

by Yvonne Canal, Community Dietitian

4 small chicken quarters, with the skin removed

30 ml / 2 tbsp lemon juice

2 tsp seasoning mix (homemade or bought)

1 medium-sized onion, sliced

2 cloves garlic, peeled and chopped

15 ml / 1 tbsp olive oil

1 small pepper, sliced (green/red/orange/yellow)

2 fresh tomatoes

½ chicken stock cube

1 bay leaf

homemade seasoning mixes:

pepper, salt and dried herbs such as thyme or oregano

1. Heat the oven to 180 degrees C or gas mark 4.
2. Wash the chicken quarters and dry with kitchen paper. Make two small slits on one side of the chicken portions. Place in a bowl.
3. Rub into the chicken the lemon juice, seasoning mix and add half of the sliced onion and garlic.
4. Cover and leave to marinate in the fridge for at least two hours.
5. Remove the chicken from the marinade and place on a wire rack in a roasting pan. Bake for 15–20 minutes until the chicken is starting to brown on top.
6. Meanwhile, start preparing the gravy by heating the oil in a pan and adding the remaining sliced onion, pepper and garlic. Cook for 2–3 minutes. Add the tomatoes and cook for a further 4 minutes.
7. Make up the stock cube with 200 ml / ⅓ pint of boiling water and add this to the pan with the bay leaf and stir well. Set aside.
8. Remove the chicken from the oven and take it off the rack. Drain off any fat from the roasting pan. Pour the gravy into the bottom of the pan and place the chicken in the pan.

9. Cover loosely with aluminium foil, place the pan back in the oven and cook for a further 45 minutes or until the chicken is cooked.

10. Remove the bay leaf before serving, and serve with potatoes and vegetables.

Tip: Bought seasoning mixes are often high in salt – it is usually listed as the first ingredient.

Per serving: energy 220 kcal, protein 28 g, fat 9 g, carbohydrate 3 g

main courses: fish

PAELLA (serves 4)

by Fernando Dieguez, Pharmacy porter

'This is a healthy low fat dish.' — Fernando

- 125 g / 4½ oz chicken breast
- 125 g / 4½ oz lean pork
- 50 g / 1¾ oz squid
- 15 ml / 1 tbsp olive oil
- 1 medium onion, finely chopped
- 2 cloves garlic, crushed
- 100 g / 3½ oz tomatoes, chopped
- 50 g / 1¾ oz pimentos
- 200 g / 7 oz rice
- 500 ml / 18 fl oz water
- 100 g / 4 oz mixed seafood
- 50 g / 1¾ oz prawns
- salt and pepper
- shelled prawns and additional pimentos for garnish

1. Dice the chicken and pork into small cubes, and cut the squid into strips.
2. Fry the chicken and pork and in the oil and when nearly cooked add the chopped onion and continue cooking until golden in colour.
3. Add the garlic, chopped tomatoes, pimentos and squid and cook for a few minutes.
4. Add the rice and continue cooking until virtually all the moisture in the pan has been absorbed.

5. Add the water and bring to the boil. Once the rice has started to thicken, add the mixed seafood and prawns and stir well.
6. Add salt and pepper to taste.
7. Turn down the heat, place a lid on the pan and continue to cook on a low heat until the rice is completely cooked.
8. Transfer to a warmed serving dish and decorate with prawns and thin strips of pimento before serving.

> Per serving: energy 320 kcals,
> protein 32 g, fat 12 g,
> carbohydrate 46 g
> Medium GI

TARRAGON STUFFED TROUT

(serves 4) *by Anne Care*

4 x trout

2 slices of crustless brown bread, made into breadcrumbs

6 sprigs of fresh tarragon (chop up 4 of them)

1 egg

1 medium-sized onion, sliced

salt and pepper

150 ml / 5 fl oz dry white wine

1. Preheat oven to 200 degrees C or gas mark 6.
2. Wash the trout and place in a non-stick baking tray.
3. In a bowl mix together the breadcrumbs, chopped tarragon, beaten egg and seasoning.
4. Stuff the trout with the breadcrumb mix.
5. Sprinkle the sliced onion over the trout.
6. Pour wine into the baking tray around the trout.
7. Cover the baking tray tightly with foil and bake in the middle of the oven for 25 minutes.
8. Serve with new potatoes and a crisp green salad.

Per serving: energy 300 kcal, protein 34 g, fat 9 g, carbohydrate 10 g

FRESH TUNA KEBABS (serves 4)

by Afizah Noobeebuy, Diabetes Specialist Nurse

fresh tuna steak, weighing 500 g / 1 lb 2 oz
juice of a lemon
1 large courgette, cut into 1.25 cm / ½ inch slices
8 cherry tomatoes
1 pepper (green or red) cut into small pieces

1. Cut the tuna into cubes. Combine with the lemon juice and chill for 30 minutes.
2. Thread the fish, courgette, tomatoes and peppers on four skewers, alternating each ingredient along the skewer.
3. Grill until the tuna and vegetables are cooked through.
4. Serve with pitta bread and a salad.

Per serving: energy 250 kcals, protein 30 g, fat 7 g, carbohydrate 3 g

MADRAS FISH CURRY (serves 4)

by Kirilee Oliver, Dietitian

'Different varieties of white fish, or oily fish like salmon or mackerel, can be used in this recipe.' – Kirilee

4 cod or haddock steaks, 150 g / 5½ oz each

1 medium onion, chopped

2.5 cm / 1 inch root ginger, chopped

2 cloves of garlic

30 ml / 2 tbsp vinegar

15 ml / 1 tbsp olive oil

½ tsp cumin seeds

½ tsp fennel seeds

½ tsp ground coriander

½ tsp turmeric

½ tsp ground cumin

2 tomatoes, chopped

1 tsp garam masala

1 tsp salt

freshly ground black pepper

200 ml / 7 fl oz water

1. Put the onion, ginger, garlic and vinegar in a food processor and blend to a smooth paste.
2. Put the oil in a large non-stick pan over a medium heat. When it is hot, add the cumin and fennel seeds and cook for around 4 minutes.
3. Pour in the paste from the food processor and fry for 10 minutes, stirring regularly.
4. Add the coriander, turmeric and cumin and continue stirring for approximately 1 minute.
5. Next add the tomatoes, garam masala, salt and freshly ground black pepper. Continue cooking for 3 minutes.

6. Stir in the water, bring to the boil, cover the pan, reduce the heat and simmer gently for about 20 minutes.

7. Place the fish in the pan making sure that each fish steak is separate from the next one, spoon the sauce mixture over the fish and simmer gently for 10 to 15 minutes until the fish is cooked through.

8. Serve with rice or nan bread and a salad.

Tip: Use a non-stick pan when cooking so you don't have to use as much oil. Try using the low calorie spray oils.

> Per serving: energy 150 kcals, protein 27 g, fat 7 g, carbohydrate 2 g

TUNA AND CORN FISHCAKES
(serves 4)

by Mercia Ross, Clerical Officer, Antenatal Clinic

300 g / 10½ oz mashed potato
200 g / 7 oz can tuna fish, drained
100 g / 3½ oz canned or frozen sweetcorn
2 tbsp chopped fresh parsley
50 g / 1¾ oz fresh white or brown breadcrumbs
salt and black pepper
lemon wedges to serve

1. Place the mashed potato in a bowl and stir in the tuna fish, sweetcorn and chopped parsley.
2. Season to taste with salt and black pepper.
3. Divide the mixture into eight, and shape into patty shapes.
4. Spread the breadcrumbs on a plate and press the fishcakes into the breadcrumbs to coat lightly. Place on a baking sheet.
5. Cook the fishcakes under a moderately hot grill until crisp and golden brown. Turn once.
6. Serve hot, with lemon wedges accompanied by a selection of vegetables or salad.

Per serving (2 fishcakes):
energy 230 kcal, protein 24 g,
fat 10 g, carbohydrate 23 g
High GI

BHUNA FISH STEAKS (serves 4)

by Lyn Pratley, Diabetes Specialist Nurse

'This recipe is quick to prepare and cook, and is low in fat.' – Lyn

4 cod steaks, 150 g / 5½ oz each
15 ml / 1 tbsp olive oil
for the marinade:
2.5 cm / 1 inch fresh root ginger, grated
2 cloves of garlic
1 tsp garam masala
½ tsp ground cumin
½ tsp turmeric
½ tsp mustard powder
15 ml / 1 tbsp lemon juice
1 tsp salt
freshly ground black pepper

1. Mix all the ingredients for the marinade in a bowl. Add 15 ml / 1 tbsp, or so, of warm water to make it into a paste.
2. Cover the fish steaks on both sides with the marinade and leave to stand for 15 minutes.
3. Line the inside of a grill pan with foil, and brush it with a little of the oil.
4. Preheat the grill.
5. Drizzle half the oil over the fish and grill for 6 minutes.
6. Turn the steaks over, drizzle the remaining oil over the fish and grill the second side for a further 5 minutes.
7. Serve with rice or naan bread and accompanied by a salad or curried vegetables.

Tip: Rather than frying foods, grill, boil, stew, steam, poach, microwave or bake them.

Per serving: energy 185 kcals, protein 26 g, fat 8.5 g, carbohydrate virtually nil

GOAN PRAWN CURRY (serves 4)

by Anne Smart, Specialist Nurse

'This recipe can be made with a lower fat content by using a low fat coconut milk rather then the standard product.' – Anne

- 15 ml / 1 tbsp paprika
- 1/2 tsp turmeric
- 2 tsp ground coriander
- 1 tsp ground cumin
- 15 ml / 1 tbsp lemon juice
- 1 tsp salt
- 1/2 tsp cayenne pepper
- 100 ml / 3 1/2 fl oz water
- 15 ml / 1 tbsp olive oil
- 1/2 tsp mustard seeds
- 1 large onion, finely sliced
- 2 cloves garlic
- 400 ml can of coconut milk
- 500 g / 1 lb 2 oz prawns (peeled)

1. Put the paprika, turmeric, coriander, cumin, lemon juice, salt, cayenne pepper and water in a bowl and mix well to form a smooth paste.
2. Put the oil in a deep frying pan over a medium heat. When hot, add the mustard seeds, onion and garlic. Cook, stirring continually, until golden brown.
3. Stir in the spice paste and bring to a simmer, then turn down the heat to low.
4. Cover and simmer gently for 10 minutes.
5. Add the coconut milk (well stirred) and prawns.
6. Continue to simmer until the prawns are cooked.
7. Serve with boiled rice.

Per serving: energy 275 kcals, protein 28 g, fat 10 g, carbohydrate 2 g

ROASTED TILAPIA OR SNAPPER

(**serves 4**) *by James Maganga, patient with Type 2 diabetes*
'This is a healthy dish; the fish is not fried and there is a good
selection of fresh vegetables to accompany the fish.' – James

> 2 medium-sized tilapia or snapper
> juice of 2 lemons
> 2 cloves of garlic
> pinch of paprika
> 4 bay leaves
> dill
> 15 ml / 1 tbsp of olive oil
> cracked pepper

1. Mix all the ingredients together to make a marinade.
2. Place the fish in a dish and cover with the marinade and place in the fridge for about 12 hours.
3. Preheat the oven to 180 degrees C, gas mark 4.
4. Place the fish in a roasting dish and cook for about 20–25 minutes until cooked through and tender.
5. Serve with potatoes and a medley of vegetables like carrots, French beans, swede and parsnips.

> Per serving: energy 250 kcals, protein 40 g, fat 7g, carbohydrate virtually nil

FISH PIE (serves 4)

500 g / 1 lb 2 oz white fish e.g. cod or haddock
300 ml / ½ pint milk
25 g / 1 oz butter
25 g / 1 oz plain flour
100 g / 3½ oz peeled prawns
2 eggs, hard boiled and cut into quarters
15 ml / 1 tbsp lemon juice
1 tbsp chopped parsley
salt and pepper
for the potato topping:
500 g / 1 lb 2 oz boiled potatoes
50 ml / 2 fl oz milk
15 g / ½ oz butter
salt and pepper
25 g / 1 oz grated cheddar cheese

1. Preheat the oven to 200 degrees C, gas mark 6.
2. Place the fish in a dish with 2 tbsp of the milk, cover with foil and bake for 20 minutes until cooked. Remove from the oven, take the skin off the fish and flake it into largish chunks. Reserve the liquid from the fish.
3. Make the sauce by melting the butter in a pan, and then stirring in the flour.
4. Gradually stir in the liquid from the cooked fish and the remaining milk, stirring continually so that the sauce does not go lumpy. Simmer for 3 minutes. Season with salt and pepper.
5. Mix the fish into the sauce, add the prawns and quartered hard-boiled eggs and parsley. Stir in the lemon juice.
6. Put the fish mixture into a lightly oiled or buttered baking dish.
7. Make the potato topping by mashing the boiled potatoes with the milk and butter (this mixes in well if the milk is warmed a little first).
8. Add salt and pepper to taste.

9. Spread the potato over the fish mixture and sprinkle the grated cheese on top.
10. Place near the top of the oven and bake for 30 minutes until the pie is hot throughout and the top will be nicely browned.

> Per serving: energy : 425 kcals, protein 39 g, fat 20 g, carbohydrate 30 g.
> High GI

GRILLED MACKEREL (serves 4)

by Kala, Pathology Department, Newham University Hospital NHS Trust

4 whole mackerel, well cleaned
2 tsp ginger paste
2 tsp garlic paste
2 tsp ground black pepper
1 tsp turmeric powder
2 tsp lemon juice
salt

1. Mix all the spices together with the lemon juice and marinate the fish. Place in the fridge for 45 minutes.
2. Preheat the oven to 190 degrees C, gas mark 5.
3. Place the mackerel in a baking dish and cook for 45 minutes.
4. Serve with rice, natural yoghurt and vegetables.

> Per serving: energy 170 kcals, protein 23 g, fat 12 g, carbohydrate nil

MAURITIAN PRAWN AND LOBSTER CURRY (serves 4)

by Vijaya Munian, Ward Clerk, Plashet Ward, Newham General Hospital

450 g / 1 lb lobster flesh (1 lobster)

15 ml / 1 tbsp olive oil

1 clove garlic, crushed

1 large onion, finely chopped

1 tsp ginger paste

1 tsp chilli powder

450 g / 1 lb prawns

2 medium-sized tomatoes

salt

coriander leaves

1. Remove the flesh from the lobster shell.
2. Heat the oil in a pan and fry the garlic and onion on a low heat until browned.
3. Add the ginger paste and chilli powder and continue to cook for 2 minutes.
4. Add the prawns and lobster to the sauce, cover and cook on a medium heat for 5 minutes.
5. Add 50 ml / 2 fl oz of water, the flesh of the tomatoes and stir carefully.
6. Cover the pan and simmer for about 15–20 minutes. Add a little salt.
7. Garnish with coriander leaves before serving.
8. Accompany this curry with rice.

> Per serving: energy 285 kcals, protein 50 g, fat 10 g, carbohydrate 1.5 g

MARINATED SALMON (serves 4)

by Barry, Newham University Hospital NHS Trust

4 salmon fillets
15 ml / 1 tbsp honey
15 ml / 1 tbsp soy sauce
2.5 cm / 1 inch piece of root ginger, finely chopped
1 clove of garlic, chopped

1. Mix the honey, soy sauce, ginger and garlic together to make the marinade.
2. Place the salmon fillets in a dish and cover with the marinade and place in the fridge for 1–2 hours.
3. Preheat the grill to a medium setting, place the salmon fillets on a baking tray and grill until cooked, turning once.
4. Serve with boiled new potatoes and green beans.

Per serving: energy 250 kcals,
protein 23 g, fat 15 g,
carbohydrate 3 g

vegetarian dishes

PASTA PROVENCALE (serves 4)

by Pauline Farlam, Staff Nurse, Plashet Ward, Newham General Hospital

225 g / 8 oz penne

15 ml / 1 tbsp olive oil

25 g / 1 oz stoned black olives, chopped

400 g can of artichoke hearts, halved

115 g / 4 oz baby plum tomatoes, halved

115 g / 4 oz courgettes, trimmed and sliced

100–115 g / 4 oz assorted young salad leaves

salt and pepper

for the dressing:

60 ml / 4 tbsp passata

30 ml / 2 tbsp natural yoghurt

15 ml / 1 tbsp unsweetened orange juice

1 small bunch of fresh basil, shredded, to garnish

1. Cook the penne in a saucepan of boiling water according to the instructions on the packet.
2. Stir in the olive oil and olives. Season with salt and pepper. Leave to cool.
3. Mix the artichokes, courgettes and plum tomatoes in with the cooked pasta.
4. Make the dressing by mixing the passata, yoghurt and orange juice together and stir in to the vegetable and pasta mixture.
5. Arrange the salad leaves in a serving bowl.
6. Spoon the pasta on top of the salad and garnish with shredded basil leaves.

> Per serving: energy 285 kcals, protein 14 g, fat 5 g, carbohydrate 50 g
> Low GI

VEGETABLE GOULASH (serves 4)

15 ml / 1 tbsp olive oil

2 medium onions

2 tsp of plain flour

1 tbsp Hungarian paprika

275 ml / 9½ fl oz hot water with 1 tsp tomato puree
dissolved in it

225 g / 8 oz cauliflower florets

225 g / 8 oz carrots, cut into chunks

225 g / 8 oz courgettes, cut into chunks

225 g / 8 oz new potatoes, cut in half

1 green pepper, chopped

400 g can tomatoes

1 tsp dried, mixed herbs

150 ml / 5 fl oz soured cream or Greek yoghurt

salt and black pepper

1. Preheat the oven to 180 degrees C, gas mark 4.
2. Heat the oil in a casserole and fry the onions until softened.
3. Stir in the flour and most of the paprika and cook for a minute.
4. Add the tomato puree and the water and bring to the boil,
   stirring continually.
5. Add all the vegetables.
6. Add the mixed herbs and season with salt and pepper.
7. Put the lid on the casserole and transfer to the oven and cook
   for 40 minutes.
8. Before serving, stir in the soured cream or yoghurt and
   sprinkle the remainder of the paprika on the top.
9. Serve with rice or noodles.

Per serving: energy 215 kcals,
protein 5 g, fat 12 g,
carbohydrate 20 g

BEAN CASSEROLE (serves 4)

by Dr Geoff Packe, Consultant Physician, Newham University Hospital NHS Trust

225 g / 8 oz dried beans e.g. haricot or flageolet
15 ml / 1 tbsp olive oil
1 medium onion, chopped
1 stick of celery, finely chopped
225 g / 8 oz carrots, sliced
200 g (small tin) plum tomatoes
4 tsp wholegrain mustard
30 ml / 2 tbsp soy sauce
1 tsp cumin powder
1 tbsp muscavado sugar
85 ml / 3 fl oz Guinness (or wine instead)

1. Soak the beans overnight.
2. Drain the beans and cook in plenty of water until tender. Drain.
3. Heat the oil in a heavy-bottomed casserole dish and cook the onion, celery and carrots for 5 minutes.
4. Then add the tomatoes, mustard, soy sauce, cumin, sugar, beans and the Guinness or wine.
5. Bring to the boil, stirring occasionally, then turn down the heat so the casserole is simmering.
6. Put the lid on the casserole and continue to cook for at least 1½ hours. Stir occasionally during the cooking, and if the beans are drying out add a little more water.
7. When cooked, all the vegetables will be tender. Adjust the seasoning before serving. This dish goes well with roasted sweet potatoes and relish.

Per serving: energy 200 kcals,
protein 13 g, fat 4 g,
carbohydrate 46 g
Low GI.

STUFFED RED PEPPERS (serves 4)

by Madhu Sharma, Dietitian, Newham University Hospital NHS Trust

4 medium-sized red peppers
1 medium aubergine, diced
100 g / 3½ oz feta cheese
3 medium tomatoes, diced
12 button mushrooms, diced
100 g / 3½ oz sliced black olives
15 ml / 1 tbsp olive oil
2 cloves garlic, crushed
2 tsp dried oregano

1. Preheat the oven to 190 degrees C, gas mark 5.
2. Cut the peppers into halves and deseed.
3. Mix together the aubergine, feta cheese, tomatoes, mushrooms and black olives and put into the pepper halves.
4. Mix together the olive oil, crushed garlic and oregano and pour over the peppers.
5. Place on a baking tray in the oven and cook for 30 minutes.
6. Serve hot with rice or pitta bread.

Per serving: energy 180 kcals, protein 28 g, fat 14 g, carbohydrate 3 g

RATATOUILLE (serves 4)

2 medium-sized aubergines
3 medium courgettes
2 medium onions
1 red pepper
1 green pepper
15 ml / 1 tbsp olive oil
2 cloves of garlic
400 g can tomatoes, drained
salt and black pepper
basil leaves, chopped

1. Cut the aubergine into slices and then into 2.5 cm / 1 inch chunks.
2. Cut the courgettes into 2.5 cm / 1 inch chunks.
3. Place both these vegetables in a colander and sprinkle with salt and allow to stand for 45 minutes. The salt will draw out the excess moisture.
4. Chop the onions and de-seed and cut up the peppers.
5. Heat the oil in a pan and fry the onions and garlic for 5 minutes or so and then add the peppers.
6. Dry the aubergine and courgettes with kitchen paper and then add to the onions, garlic and peppers.
7. Add the drained tinned tomatoes.
8. Season with salt and pepper and chopped basil.
9. Simmer gently, uncovered, for about 20–30 minutes until the vegetables are cooked but not mushy. Serve with rice.

Tip: This dish is an excellent way to use up surplus vegetables at the end of the summer when the harvest is plentiful and prices low. It can also be pureed in a blender to make a delicious soup.

Per serving: energy 75 kcals, protein 7.5 g, fat 4 g, carbohydrate 8.4 g

SPINACH & OKRA CURRY (serves 4)

by Sheila Ryan, Lead Nurse in Cardiac Rehabilitation

'Spinach is a good dietary source of iron. This is a great interesting recipe using spinach and okra.' — *Sheila*

> 250 g / 9 oz spinach
> 15 ml / 1 tbsp olive oil
> 1 hot red chilli
> ½ onion, sliced
> 250 g / 9 oz okra, sliced
> ½ tsp salt
> ½ tsp garam masala
> 30 ml / 2 tbsp single cream

1. Wash and chop the spinach leaves.
2. Heat the oil in a large frying pan or wok, add the chilli and stir until darkened.
3. Add the onion and stir until browned.
4. Add the okra, salt and garam masala. Stir well and cook for 5 minutes.
5. Then add the spinach and cook until it has wilted.
6. Add the cream and cook, stirring regularly, for a further 4 minutes.
7. Serve with rice or nan bread.

Per serving: energy 40 kcals, protein 3 g, fat 2 g, carbohydrate 3 g

LENTIL MOUSSAKA (serves 4)

This is a delicious non-meat version of a classic Greek dish

100 g / 3½ oz green lentils
225 ml / 8 fl oz water
2 medium-sized aubergines
15 ml / 1 tbsp olive oil
2 cloves of garlic
2 medium onions
2 green peppers
4 button mushrooms, sliced
15 ml / 1 tbsp tomato puree
½ tsp ground cinnamon
1 tbsp chopped parsley
125 ml / 4 fl oz red wine
salt and black pepper
for the topping:
1 medium egg
150 ml / 5 fl oz natural yoghurt
grated nutmeg
50 g / 1¾ oz grated mature cheese e.g. cheddar

1. Preheat the oven to 180 degrees C, gas mark 4.
2. Lightly oil a large ovenproof dish.
3. Cook the lentils gently in the water until softened (about 30 minutes).
4. Slice the aubergines to a thickness of about 1 cm / ½ inch and place the slices in a colander and sprinkle with salt. Leave to stand for about 20 minutes so that the excess moisture is drawn out of the aubergine. When ready to use, wipe the aubergine slices dry with kitchen paper.
5. Meanwhile, heat half the oil in a non-stick frying pan and cook the garlic, onions and peppers for 5 minutes until softened.
6. Add the sliced mushrooms and continue cooking for 5 minutes.

7. Put all the vegetables to one side.
8. Add the remainder of the oil to the pan and fry the aubergines for about 10 minutes, turning once, then put to one side.
9. Mix the tomato puree, cinnamon, salt, pepper, parsley and wine together in a jug and pour this into the vegetable mixture. Stir in the lentils.
10. Place a layer of sliced aubergine in the ovenproof dish and then cover with a layer of lentil and vegetable mix. Repeat this, finishing with a layer of aubergine.
11. Beat the egg into the yoghurt, add a little nutmeg and the grated cheese. Pour on top of the aubergine and lentils.
12. Bake for about 30 minutes until the top is golden brown.
13. Serve accompanied with pitta bread or rice.

Per serving: energy 215 kcals, protein 10 g, fat 14 g, carbohydrate 10 g
Low GI

SPINACH AND RICOTTA LASAGNE (serves 4)

500 g / 1 lb 2 oz frozen spinach

15 ml / 1 tbsp olive oil

1 clove garlic, crushed

2 medium-sized onions, chopped

400 g tin of chopped tomatoes

8 button mushrooms, sliced

1 tsp dried mixed herbs

9 lasagne sheets

salt and pepper

250 g / 9 oz tub of ricotta cheese

for the sauce:

40 g / 1½ oz butter

25 g / 1 oz plain flour

425 ml / ¾ pint semi-skimmed milk

25 g / 1 oz grated Cheddar cheese

1. Preheat the oven to 180 degrees C, gas mark 4.
2. Boil the spinach for 5 minutes until cooked, and then drain well.
3. Heat the oil in a pan and cook the garlic and onion for 5 minutes until soft.
4. Add the tomatoes and mushrooms, mixed herbs, salt and pepper.
5. To make the sauce, melt the butter in a pan and stir in the flour.
6. Add the milk slowly, stirring continually.
7. Lightly oil an ovenproof dish measuring approximately 18 x 24 cm (7 x 9½ inches).
8. Place three sheets of lasagne on the bottom of the dish. Cover with half the drained spinach and half the tomato and onion mixture. Then put the ricotta cheese on top, spooned out of the tub in small pieces.
9. Cover with another layer of lasagne sheets, the remaining

spinach and tomato/onion mixture and finish with the remaining three lasagne sheets.

10. Pour the white sauce over the top of the lasagne and sprinkle with the grated cheese. Bake in the oven for 40 minutes.

> Per serving: energy 580 kcals, protein 30 g, fat 26 g, carbohydrate 65 g
> Low GI

VEGETABLE CURRY (serves 4)

by Harpreet Kaur, Health Advocate and wife of a person with diabetes

> 2 large carrots, sliced
> 300 ml / ½ pint vegetable stock
> 1 onion, sliced
> 1 small cauliflower
> 2 courgettes, sliced
> 2 tomatoes, quartered
> 15 ml / 1 tbsp curry paste
> 30 ml / 2 tbsp lime juice
> 2 hard-boiled eggs, quartered

1. Place the carrots in a saucepan with the vegetable stock, bring to the boil, cover and simmer for 10 minutes.
2. Add the onion, cauliflower, courgettes, tomatoes, curry paste and lime juice.
3. Cover and simmer for 10 minutes until the vegetables are just tender.
4. Decorate with quartered hard boiled egg.
5. Serve with boiled rice or nan bread.

> Per serving: energy 55 kcals, protein 4 g, fat 3g, carbohydrate 5 g

WILD MUSHROOM RISOTTO
(serves 4)

   40 g / 1½ oz dried porcini mushrooms
   450 g / 1 lb mixed fresh mushrooms including wild varieties
       like chanterelles and girolles (halve any mushrooms that
       are large)
   15 ml / 1 tbsp olive oil
   2 cloves of garlic, crushed
   1 medium onion, finely chopped
   250 g/ 9 oz Arborio rice
   100 ml / 3½ fl oz dry white wine
   700 ml / 1¼ pints chicken stock
   25 g / 1 oz freshly grated Parmesan cheese
   salt and pepper
   3 tbsp chopped parsley

1. Place the dried mushrooms in a small bowl and pour over
    boiling water to cover them. Leave to soak for 30 minutes,
    then lift them out and pat them dry.
2. Strain the liquor from the mushrooms and reserve this to use
    later.
3. Trim the fresh mushrooms and brush clean.
4. Heat half the oil in a non-stick pan over a low heat, add the
    mushrooms and fry for 2 minutes.
5. Add the garlic and soaked mushrooms and cook, stirring, for
    another 2 minutes. Transfer to a plate and reserve.
6. Heat the remaining oil in a large saucepan, add the onion and
    cook for 2 minutes until softened.
7. Add the rice and cook until translucent. Stir frequently.
8. Add the wine, and when it is almost absorbed add a ladleful of
    the stock. Continue to cook, stirring, until the liquid is absorbed.
9. Continue to add the stock, a ladleful at a time allowing each
    addition to become absorbed before adding the next. This will

take about 20 minutes. The rice should be of creamy consistency but still firm to the bite.

10. Add half the reserved mushroom soaking liquid to the risotto and stir in the mushrooms. Season to taste with salt and pepper.

11. Remove from the heat and stir in the Parmesan cheese and most of the chopped parsley.

12. Transfer into warmed serving bowls and garnish with the remainder of the parsley.

> Per serving: energy 311 kcals, protein 8 g, fat 7 g, carbohydrate 54 g
> High GI

EGG BIRYANI (serves 4)

by Edna Smith, PA in Nursing

15 ml / 1 tbsp olive oil

6 black peppercorns

2 green cardamom

5 cm / 2 inch cinnamon stick

1 tsp cumin seeds

2 bay leaves

1 medium onion, sliced

2 cloves of garlic

1 cm / ½ inch root ginger

1 green chilli, chopped

1 tsp red chilli powder

1 tsp coriander powder

1 tsp garam masala

1 tsp salt

200 g / 7 oz basmati rice

400 ml / 14 fl oz water

4 eggs (hard boiled)

coriander leaves to garnish

1. Heat the oil in a non-stick pan. Add the peppercorns, cardamom, cinnamon, cumin seeds, and bay leaves and fry for 1 minute. Then reduce the heat.

2. Add the sliced onion, garlic, ginger and green chilli; fry until golden brown.

3. Add the red chilli powder, coriander powder, garam masala and salt.

4. Add the rice and water, stir well, cover and cook for 20 minutes on a medium heat.

5. Meanwhile slice the hard-boiled eggs and arrange around the edge of a serving dish.

6. Place the rice in the middle of the dish and garnish with coriander leaves.

Per serving: energy 214 kcals, protein 6.5 g, fat 9.7 g, carbohydrate 30 g

Medium GI

SAFFRON RICE (serves 4)

by Vania Barbara, trainee surgical care practitioner in orthopaedics, Newham University Hospital NHS Trust

> 15 ml / 1 tbsp olive oil
> 200 g / 7 oz Arborio rice
> 4 strands of saffron
> 75 ml / ½ glass of dry white wine
> 500 ml / 18 fl oz vegetable stock
> 25 g / 1 oz of grated Parmesan cheese
> salt and pepper

1. Heat the olive oil in a pan on a medium heat.
2. Add the rice and stir. Lower the heat.
3. Add the saffron and wine.
4. Stir occasionally for a few minutes and then add the vegetable stock gradually. Add a ladleful of stock at a time and wait until the rice has absorbed the previous quantity of stock before adding the next one.
5. Add ¾ of the Parmesan cheese, a little salt and black pepper.
6. When the rice is 'al dente' i.e. still has a bite to it, switch off the heat.
7. Dish up the rice between four serving plates and sprinkle the remaining Parmesan over the top before serving.

Per serving: energy 250 kcals, protein 5.5 g, fat 6 g, carbohydrate 44 g
High GI

DHAL (serves 4)

by Hayley Kuter, Dietitian

'As a vegetarian, I often use lentil recipes. Dhal is quick to prepare, and it's very nutritious.' – Hayley

- 75 g / 2¾ oz mung dhal (yellow split peas)
- 75 g / 2¾ oz masoor dhal (red lentils)
- ½ tsp ground turmeric
- 850 ml / 1½ pints water
- 1½ tsp salt
- 15 ml / 1 tbsp olive oil
- ½ tsp cumin seeds
- 2 hot red chillies
- 1 clove of garlic, crushed

1. Put the dhals in a bowl of water and wash in two changes of water.
2. Place the dhals in a saucepan and add the turmeric and water.
3. Bring to the boil over a medium heat and then turn down the heat.
4. Partly cover the pan and simmer gently over a low heat for about 40 minutes until the dhals are very soft.
5. Stir in the salt. Turn off the heat and place the lid on the saucepan.
6. In a small frying pan, heat the oil and add the cumin seeds and chillies.
7. Once the chillies have darkened (which happens very quickly) add the garlic and brown.
8. When the garlic has cooked, pour the spices in the frying pan onto the dhals and replace the lid on the saucepan.
9. Serve with rice and nan.

> Per serving: energy 120 kcals, protein 8 g, fat 4 g, carbohydrate 13 g
> Low GI

SAVOURY CARIBBEAN RICE (serves 4)

by Yvonne Canal, Community Dietitian

'This dish is quick to prepare. The vegetables that you use can also be varied. It can be used to accompany meat, poultry, or fish dishes either of European or Oriental origin.' — Yvonne

> 200 g / 7 oz rice (brown, white or basmati)
> stock cube of your choice
> 150 g / 5½ oz of mixed vegetables e.g. peas, sweetcorn,
>   carrots

1. Place the rice in a large microwave container with a lid.
2. Measure out 400 ml of boiling water and dissolve the stock cube in it.
3. Add the vegetables to the rice and then pour on the stock. Stir.
4. Put the lid on and cook for 14 minutes in the microwave on a medium–medium-high setting.
5. Remove the container from the microwave and allow to stand for 2 minutes, then remove the lid and stir.
6. Taste the rice to see if it is fully cooked; if not add 1–2 tbsp (15–30 ml of hot water), replace the lid and cook for a further 1–2 minutes.
7. If the rice is too wet at the end of the cooking time, place it back in the microwave and cook for a further 1–2 minutes but do not add any additional water.

Tip: Be careful when removing a container from a microwave oven and taking the lid off as a lot of steam can be generated during the cooking process.

> Per serving: energy 200 kcals,
> protein 5 g, fat 0.5 g,
> carbohydrate 50 g

MOROCCAN VEGETABLE COUSCOUS (serves 4 as a main meal, 8 as a snack)

By Jennifer Swan, HIV Specialist Pharmacist, Newham University Hospital NHS Trust

For the vegetable selection:
6 cloves of garlic, roughly chopped
3 red or white onions, sliced
6 peppers, sliced
4 medium courgettes, sliced
15 ml / 1 tbsp olive oil
salt and black pepper
(For variety, the onions, peppers and courgettes could be swapped for shallots, an aubergine, 3 parboiled and lengthwise sliced carrots, 3 parboiled and lengthwise sliced parsnips.)

for the couscous:
360 g / 12¼ oz couscous
1 vegetable stock cube (optional)
juice of one lemon

for the sauce:
15 ml / 1 tbsp tomato puree
1 tsp cumin
juice of 1 lemon
15 ml / 1 tbsp balsamic vinegar

1. Preheat the oven to 180 degrees C, gas mark 4.
2. Place the sliced and chopped vegetables on a baking tray.
3. Pour the olive oil over the vegetables and add a pinch of salt and black pepper. Add 30 ml / 2 tbsp of water.
4. Place in the oven and roast for an hour, tossing them halfway through and adding an additional 15 ml / 1 tbsp of water
5. Make up the couscous as per instructions on the packet. Use either stock or hot water. Add the juice of a lemon.
6. Make the sauce by placing all the ingredients in a small bowl and mixing well. Add extra water if the sauce is too thick.

7. Assemble the dish by placing the couscous on a serving dish, covering with the roasted vegetables and finally drizzling the sauce over the top.

> Per serving: energy 410 kcals,
> protein 11 g, fat 6 g,
> carbohydrate 77 g
> High GI

PUNJABI MUNG CURRY (serves 4)

by Dr Shanti Vijayaraghavan, Consultant Physician, Newham University Hospital NHS Trust

> 200 g / 7 oz mung dhal (yellow split peas)
> 100 g / 3½ oz onion, chopped
> 2 tsp olive oil
> 200 g can tomatoes
> 1 clove garlic
> 1 cm / ½ inch finely chopped ginger
> 1 tsp coriander powder
> ½ tsp chilli powder
> 1 tsp salt

1. Wash and soak the mung for an hour.
2. Place in a saucepan and cover with plenty of water.
3. Boil for around 30 minutes (until cooked) and set aside.
4. Fry the onions until soft.
5. Add the tomatoes and spices and cook until blended together.
6. Add the mung dhal to the tomato and spice mixture and cook on a low heat for 5 to 10 minutes until heated through.
7. Serve with rice or nan bread.

> Per serving: energy 115 kcals,
> protein 9 g, fat 3 g,
> carbohydrate 15 g
> Low GI

snacks

SOCCA (serves 6)

by Julie Ballero, a friend of Diana's and a resident of Nice

'This is a Nicoise speciality. It makes a nice quick lunch served with a salad.' – Julie

> 500 ml / 18 fl oz of water
> 20 ml / 4 tsp of olive oil
> 250 g / 9 oz chickpea flour
> salt and pepper

1. Preheat the oven to 240 degrees C, gas mark 9.
2. Pour the water and olive oil into a large bowl.
3. Add the flour, beating continuously to form a paste and avoid lumps developing. (If the mixture does go lumpy then you can sieve it to obtain a smooth liquid paste.)
4. Season with salt and pepper.
5. Oil a straight-sided baking dish and spread the paste very thinly to a thickness of 3 mm / ⅛ inch.
6. Place the baking dish in the oven and cook for 15 minutes until well coloured – almost burned.
7. Remove from the oven and grind some fresh black pepper over the socca.
8. Cut into portions and serve hot.

> Per serving: energy 245 kcals,
> protein 12.5 g, fat 8 g,
> carbohydrate 30 g
> Low GI

POACHED EGGS AND SPINACH
(serves 4)

by Harpreet Kaur, Bilingual Health Advocate, Newham University Hospital Trust
'This dish makes an ideal light lunch.' – Harpreet

> 500 g / 1lb 2 oz spinach, washed and chopped
> 8 tbsp water
> 4 medium tomatoes
> 4 medium eggs
> salt and pepper

1. Using a non-stick pan, cook the spinach in the water for a few minutes.
2. Slice the tomatoes into rings and arrange on top of the spinach.
3. Crack the eggs on top.
4. Place the lid on the pan and continue to cook for a few minutes on a low heat until the eggs are cooked.
5. Season with a little salt and black pepper according to taste.
6. Serve on toasted wholemeal or multi-grain bread.

Tip: Frozen spinach is a convenient alternative to fresh spinach.

> Per serving (excluding the toast):
> energy 120 kcals, protein 13 g,
> fat 6 g, carbohydrate 3 g

SAMOSAS (makes 12)

Recipe donated by a member of staff (anonymous)

500 g / 1 lb 2 oz potatoes, cut into small cubes

45 ml / 3 tbsp olive oil

1 large onion, chopped

125 g / 4½ oz frozen peas or other frozen mixed vegetables

1 tsp salt

1 tsp garam masala

1 green chilli, finely chopped

125 g / 4½ oz plain flour, sieved

15 g / ½ oz margarine (olive or sunflower oil based varieties)

30 ml / 2 tbsp milk, warmed

cold water

1. Boil the cubed potato pieces until only slightly hard.
2. Heat 15 ml / 1 tbsp of the oil in a frying pan and add the chopped onion. Cook until golden.
3. Add the frozen peas or mixed vegetables and cook for 5 minutes.
4. Add the salt, garam masala and chilli and then the potatoes.
5. Cook for 2 to 3 minutes and then remove from the heat.
6. In a mixing bowl, place the sieved flour, a pinch of salt and the margarine and mix to a soft dough by gradually adding some of the warm milk.
7. Break off a little of the dough, shape it into a ball and roll it out as thin as possible into a circle the size of a saucer. Cut the circle in half.
8. Place a tablespoon of the potato and vegetable mix on one half of the semicircle of dough mix and then fold over the dough, paste the edges with milk or water and close them tightly.
9. Gently shallow fry the samosas in the remaining oil and, when golden brown on both sides, remove from the pan and place on kitchen paper to absorb any excess fat.

10. Serve warm with mint chutney.

Tip: High fat snack foods should be limited. Examples include: crisps, nuts, chevda, sev, samosas, pakoras and pastries.

> Per samosa: energy 120 kcal,
> protein 2 g, fat 4 g,
> carbohydrate 24 g
> High GI

BREAKFAST SMOOTHIE (serves 4)

by Anna Collard, Facilitator diabetes storytelling group, Newham General Hospital
'This is a delicious and healthy alternative to a standard breakfast.' – Anna

30 ml / 2 tbsp low fat yoghurt
1 tbsp rolled oats
1 medium-sized banana, peeled and chopped
kiwi fruit, peeled and chopped
medium-sized pear, peeled and chopped
4–6 strawberries
2 tsp sunflower or pumpkin seeds

1. Put all the ingredients into a blender and puree.
2. Divide between four bowls.

> Per serving: energy 80 kcals,
> protein 2 g, fat 2 g,
> carbohydrate 68 g
> Low GI

TOMATO & CAPER BRUSCHETTA
(10 slices)

400 g can whole tomatoes
2 tbsp rinsed capers
1 clove of garlic, crushed
2 tsp olive oil
1 loaf of bruschetta bread
basil leaves
rock salt and black pepper

1. Halve the tomatoes and place in a saucepan with the capers, crushed garlic and olive oil.
2. Simmer until thick.
3. Slice the bruschetta into 10 and place under a medium grill until lightly browned.
4. Tear some basil leaves and place on the slices of toasted bruschetta.
5. Spoon the tomato mixture onto each slice of bruschetta and season with freshly ground black pepper and a little rock salt.

Per slice: energy 115 kcals, protein 7.5 g, fat 2.5 g, carbohydrate 20 g

desserts

FRESH FRUIT SALAD (serves 4)

by Diana Markham, Dietitian

'Select fruit that's not overripe in order to keep the GI value of this lovely dessert in the medium rather than high range.' – Diana

> 1 medium-sized apple
> 1 small banana
> 1 medium-sized orange
> 1 small mango
> 1 kiwi fruit
> 30 ml / 1 fl oz of natural orange juice

1. Wash the apple, and then cut into quarters and chop up into small pieces.
2. Peel and cut up the banana, orange, mango and kiwi fruit.
3. Place all the fruit in a bowl and cover with the orange juice.
4. Chill in the fridge before serving.
5. Fruit salad is delicious served with low fat crème fraiche or natural yoghurt.

Tip: You can eat a 'portion' of fruit that fits in the palm of your hand, i.e. 10–12 grapes, 2 plums, 1 apple/orange, 1 medium-sized banana.

Per serving: energy 70 kcals, protein 1 g, fat nil, carbohydrate 16 g
Medium GI

FRUIT FLAVOURED MOUSSE*

(serves 4)

by Jo Stones, ESR Project Administrator, Newham University Hospital NHS Trust and daughter of a person with diabetes

'This recipe is a family favourite – it is quick, easy to make, low in sugar and fat and cheap!' – Jo

> **1 sachet of sugar free jelly crystals (any flavour of your choice but the citrus flavours are best for a real zing!)**
> **250 g tub of low fat fromage frais**

1. Make up the sachet of jelly using hot water but only use half the recommended amount on the instructions, i.e. ¼ pint rather than ½ pint.
2. Stir until the jelly crystals are dissolved.
3. Top up the jelly liquid with very cold water to the ½ pint mark in a jug.
4. Pour the jelly liquid into a large bowl and stir in the fromage frais until it is all well mixed.
5. Transfer into a serving bowl, or four individual sundae dishes, and place in the fridge for an hour or so until the mix is set.
6. Serve on its own or topped with fresh fruit.

* Only eat after a carbohydrate rich meal.

> Per serving: energy 50 kcals, protein 5 g, fat 0.5 g, carbohydrate virtually nil

PEACHES WITH MASCARPONE
(serves 4)

4 firm, ripe peaches
175 g / 6 oz mascarpone cheese
40 g / 1½ oz chopped walnuts
1 tsp oil
15 ml / 1 tbsp maple syrup

1. Cut the peaches in half and remove the stones.
2. Mix the mascarpone cheese and walnuts together in a small bowl. Chill in the fridge until required.
3. Brush the peaches with a little oil and place under a preheated medium grill for about 8 minutes, turning once.
4. Transfer the peaches to a serving dish and top with the mascarpone cheese and nut mixture.
5. Drizzle a little maple syrup over the peaches and serve immediately.

Tip: the peaches can be cooked over a barbeque if you wish.

Per serving: energy 250 kcals,
protein 7 g, fat 19 g,
carbohydrate 18 g
Low GI

DRIED FRUIT SALAD WITH YOGHURT (serves 4)

50 g / 1¾ oz dried stoned prunes
50 g / 1¾ oz dried apricots
50 g / 1¾ oz dried apples
50 g / 1¾ oz dried figs (remove the stalk ends)
grated rind and juice of an orange
50 g / 1¾ oz raisins
200 g / 7 oz low fat natural yoghurt
sprinkling of ground cinnamon to garnish
Note: you can also use Greek style yoghurt instead of natural yoghurt, and swap the orange for a lemon.

1. The day before you want to make this dessert, place the prunes, apricots, apples and figs in a large bowl and cover with 300 ml / ½ pint of cold water and leave to soak overnight.
2. The next day place the fruits in a saucepan, cover and bring to the boil and then gently simmer for 10 minutes until the fruit feels soft when tested with a skewer.
3. Turn off the heat and pour in the orange juice and grated rind. Add the raisins.
4. Place the fruit salad in a bowl to cool.
5. To serve, divide the fruit salad between four glass dishes, top with the yoghurt and sprinkle a little cinnamon on the top.

Per serving: energy 135 kcals, protein 4 g, fat 0.5 g, carbohydrate 30 g
Medium GI

WHOLEWHEAT SCONES (makes 8)

150 g / 5½ oz wholewheat flour
½ tsp ground cinnamon
2 tsp baking powder
25 g / 1 oz sugar
25 g / 1 oz margarine
40 g / 1½ oz sultanas
1 egg
45 ml / 3 tbsp milk
Note: If you want a lighter scone you can use half
wholewheat flour and half white flour.

1. Preheat the oven to 220 degrees C / gas mark 7.
2. Grease a baking tray.
3. Sift the flour, cinnamon and baking powder into a bowl. Add
   the bran remaining in the sieve. Add the sugar.
4. Rub in the margarine with your fingers until the mixture is
   crumbly. Stir in the sultanas
5. In a separate bowl beat the egg and 2 tbsp of milk.
6. Add this to the mixing bowl ingredients and mix well to form a
   soft dough which leaves the side of the bowl clean. Add a little
   extra milk if the dough is too dry.
7. Roll the dough onto a floured surface to a thickness of 2 cm /
   ¾ inch.
8. Use a 5 cm / 2 inch cutter to cut out eight scones.
9. Place on the baking tray, brush the tops with the remaining
   milk and then bake on a high shelf in the oven for 15–20
   minutes.
10. Remove from the oven and
    cool on a wire tray.

Per serving: energy: 130 kcals,
protein 3 g, fat 3.5 g,
carbohydrate 19 g
High GI

RHUBARB AND ORANGE CRUMBLE (serves 4)

by Liz Killick, Assistant Hotel Services Manager,

Newham University Hospital NHS Trust

'By using a granular sweetener rather than sugar in this recipe, the energy and carbohydrate content can be significantly reduced.' – Liz

for the crumble topping:
100 g / 3½ oz porridge oats
50 g / 1¾ oz self raising wholemeal flour
grated rind of 1 orange
100 g / 3½ oz butter or margarine
75 g / 2¾ oz soft brown sugar
for the filling:
4 long stalks / 6 smaller ones of rhubarb, cut into 2 cm /
 ¾ inch pieces
1 tbsp flour
50 g / 1¾ oz granulated sugar
juice from 1 orange

1. Preheat the oven to 190 degrees C, gas mark 5.
2. Weigh out the porridge oats and flour and put in a bowl with the orange rind.
3. Cut the butter or margarine into small pieces and rub it in to the oats and flour.
4. Add the brown sugar.
5. Combine the rhubarb with a tablespoon of flour, sugar and orange juice.
6. Arrange in a pie dish. Spread the crumble mixture on top. Bake in the oven for 45 minutes.
7. Serve warm with cream, low fat crème fraiche or custard.

Per serving: energy 460 kcals (340 kcals if sweetener used), protein 5 g, fat 23 g, carbohydrate 60 g (30 g if sweetener used)

SEMOLINA PUDDING WITH CARROTS (serves 4)

by Harpreet Kaur, Bilingual Health Advocate

'This delicious dessert does not have any added sugar in the recipe, which makes it a wonderful choice for people with diabetes.' – Harpreet

75 g / 2¾ oz semolina

600 ml / 1 pint semi-skimmed milk

½ tsp crushed cardamom

50 g / 1¾ oz carrots, finely grated

15 sultanas

1. Soak the semolina in a little of the milk and set this aside.
2. Put the remainder of the milk in a non-stick pan with the cardamom and the grated carrot, bring to the boil and cook for 10 minutes over a low heat.
3. Add the semolina mix and cook until creamy, stirring regularly and then add the sultanas.
4. Serve hot or cold.

Tip: Choose low fat options of dairy foods like milk, cheese and yoghurt.

Per serving: energy 150 kcals, protein 7 g, fat 3 g, carbohydrate 24 g

BANANA AND LIME CAKE
(makes 16 slices)

300 g / 10½ oz plain flour
2 tsp baking powder
175 g / 6 oz light muscovado sugar
grated rind of one lime
1 egg, beaten
1 banana, mashed with the juice of the lime
150 ml / 5 fl oz low-fat natural yoghurt or fromage frais
115 g / 4 oz sultanas
margarine for greasing the cake tin

1. Preheat the oven to 180 degrees C, gas mark 4.
2. Grease and line two 20 x 13 cm / 8 x 5 in loaf tins with baking paper.
3. Sift the flour and baking powder into a large mixing bowl and stir in the sugar and lime rind.
4. Make a well in the centre of the dry ingredients and add the beaten egg, mashed banana, yoghurt or fromage frais, and sultanas. Mix well.
5. Spoon the mixture into the prepared tin and level the surface. Bake for 35 to 40 minutes until firm to the touch and a skewer inserted into the centre comes out clean.
6. Let the cake cool for 10 minutes in the tin and then turn out onto a wire rack to cool completely.

Tip: You can use a larger 2 lb loaf tin and make one cake instead of two smaller ones. In this instance increase the baking time to 40 to 45 minutes

Per serving: energy 145 kcals,
protein 3.5 g, fat 1 g,
carbohydrate 32 g
High GI

KHIR (serves 4)

600 ml / 20 fl oz semi-skimmed milk
75 g / 2¾ oz basmati rice, well washed
10 almonds, blanched and thinly sliced
½ tsp crushed cardamom seeds
powdered artificial sweetener (e.g. Splenda) equivalent to
    75 g / 2¾ oz sugar
2 tsp rosewater (optional)

1. Pour the milk into a large heavy-bottomed saucepan and bring it to the boil.
2. Add the rice, stir well and keep boiling on a low heat for 30 to 40 minutes. Stir regularly to prevent the sides and bottom sticking.
3. Add the thinly sliced almonds and crushed cardamom seeds.
4. Either place the khir in a moderate oven for 30 minutes to finish cooking, or continue boiling for a further 10 to 15 minutes until it has a thick consistency.
5. At the end of cooking, add the artificial sweetener and stir well.
6. Transfer the khir to a dish and when it has cooled a little, rosewater may be mixed in if desired.

Tip: There are a wide range of low sugar desserts available e.g. 'diet' or 'lite' yoghurts and mousses, sugar free jelly, instant whip and custard mixes and low sugar rice pudding.

Per serving: energy 180 kcals,
protei n 7 g, fat 4 g,
carbohydrate 23 g
Medium GI

CARROT HALVA* (serves 4)

by Yvonne Canal, Dietitian

'Halva is a very popular dessert amongst Asian families. This recipe is made healthier than the traditional version by using skimmed milk and artificial sweetener.' – Yvonne

400 g / 14 oz carrots, peeled and grated
400 ml / 14 fl oz skimmed milk
15 g / ½ oz olive or sunflower oil margarine
¼ tsp saffron
1 tsp cardamom powder
6 almonds, chopped
powdered artificial sweetener (e.g. Splenda) equivalent to
    50 g / 1¾ oz sugar
1 tsp sliced pistachio nuts

1. Place the grated carrots and milk in a non-stick pan and cook partly covered over a low heat for about an hour or until the milk has evaporated.
2. Add the margarine, saffron, cardamom powder and chopped almonds.
3. Finally stir in the artificial sweetener.
4. Place in a serving dish and decorate with sliced pistachio nuts.
5. Can be served warm or cold.

Tip: Use low fat yoghurt, fromage frais or crème fraiche as an alternative to cream with desserts or in cooking.

* Only eat after a carbohydrate rich meal.

> Per serving: energy 110 kcals, protein 5 g, fat 5 g, carbohydrate 10 g
> Medium GI

CHOCOLATE RUM MOUSSE (serves 4)

200 g / 7 oz plain chocolate
25 g / 1 oz caster sugar
25 g / 1 oz butter
4 eggs, separated
30 ml / 2 tbsp rum

1. Break the chocolate into squares and place in a saucepan over a pan containing boiling water ('*au* bain-marie').
2. Add the sugar and butter to the chocolate and stir the mixture until all the chocolate has melted.
3. Turn off the heat.
4. Allow the melted chocolate mixture to cool for a few minutes and then add the egg yolks one by one, stirring them in well.
5. Beat the egg whites until stiff.
6. Add the rum to the chocolate mixture and then gradually fold this into the beaten egg whites using a metal spoon.
7. Pour into individual sundae dishes or ramekins.
8. Place in the fridge for about 2 hours to cool before serving.

Tip: The carbohydrate content can be reduced by using a powdered sweetener rather than caster sugar. Add this after the chocolate and butter have been melted.

Per serving: energy 425 kcals, protein 8.5 g, fat 25 g, carbohydrate 39 g
If using sweetener instead of sugar, the energy content is reduced to 400 kcals and carbohydrate to 33 g per serving.
Medium GI

who is going to support me with my diabetes?

by Anne Claydon, Diabetes Special Nurse, Newham General Hospital

When you were first told that you had diabetes I am sure that you felt isolated and afraid. But remember, you are far from being alone! There are so many people out there to help you. Most importantly, you should work in partnership with your NHS Diabetes Team and feel that you are a member of it.

YOUR ANNUAL REVIEW

Everybody with diabetes is entitled to have a specialist check-up – or 'annual review' – every year. Some general practitioners carry out these examinations or you may be sent to a Diabetes Centre to see a specialist. At your annual review:

- Discuss your diabetes control and blood sugar levels.
- Your blood sugar should be checked and results discussed.
- Blood and urine tests will be taken to see how your kidneys are working. These are usually carried out before the consultation so that the results are available for discussion.
- A blood test will be done to determine your cholesterol level and the results will be explained.
- You will be advised to visit somebody who will take a photograph of your eyes.
- Your legs and feet will be examined to check for any nerve and circulation damage.

- Your weight will be recorded.
- A general discussion should take place about how you are coping with diabetes.

YOUR DIABETES CENTRE

Every Diabetes Centre has different approaches but your basic health care should include:

- Initial and continuing education for you and your family. This is usually done by specialist nurses, dietitians and podiatrists.
- A treatment plan and goals should be negotiated between you and your health care professional.
- Regular checks on your blood sugar control and general health.

YOUR DIABETES TEAM

Your 'Diabetes Team', who will help you with your condition, will include:

- **Your General Practitioner.** He/she will have day-to-day care of you and will refer you to a specialist as needs be.
- **Practice Nurse.** These are nurses that work with your General Practitioner. Many of them run their own diabetes clinic and will look after your day to day needs.
- **Diabetes Specialist Nurse.** These are experienced general nurses who have special experience in diabetes and work only with people with diabetes.
- **Diabeteologist.** A hospital consultant who specialises in diabetes.
- **Dietitian.** Your dietitian will help you adapt your diet to make it as healthy as possible. He/she will also help keep your diabetes under control.
- **Podiatrist.** Foot specialist. You can be referred to the podiatrist by your doctor or your diabetes specialist nurse. Some have a self referral system.

- Optometrist. Eye specialist to take a photograph of your eyes and examine them to see if you have any problems. This should be done yearly.

❑ Support Groups

As well as the health professionals, support is available from your local support group. Ask your practice nurse where your local team meet, and when. These groups are invaluable as people with diabetes give and receive support to each other. The best thing is, they know what you are going through!

Diabetes UK: A charity dedicated to diabetes, offering many services and lots of advice about diabetes care. A magazine, called *Balance*, is sent to all its members. *Balance* is full of useful tips and articles and looks at recent research. Diabetes UK also has a care line (0845 120 2960) that you can contact if you have a problem or a query about diabetes. I recommend that all my patients join this organisation. Further information about Diabetes UK can be found at http://www.diabetes.org.uk.

Whatever you do, remember that if you have diabetes, you are not alone! There are lots of people out there who are eager to help you.

useful contacts

Alcohol Concern
64 Leman Street
London
E1 8EU
Tel: 020 7264 0510
www.alcoholconcern.org.uk

British Heart Foundation
14 Fitzhardinge Street
London
W1H 6DH
Tel: 020 7935 0185
www.bhf.org.uk

Diabetes UK
Macleod House
10 ParkwayLondon
NW1 7AA
Tel: 020 7424 1000
www.diabetes.org.uk

Driver and Vehicle Licensing
Agency (DVLA)
DVLA Swansea
SA6 7JL
Tel: 0870 240 0009
www.dvla.gov.uk

Everydaysport
Sport England
3rd Floor Victoria House
Bloomsbury Square
London
WC1B 4SE
Tel: 020 7273 1551
www.everydaysport.com

Go Smokefree
NHS Smoking Helpline
Tel: 0800 022 4 332
www.gosmokefree.nhs.uk

National Obesity Forum
First Floor
6a Gordon Road
Nottingham
NG2 5LN
Tel: 0115 846 2109
www.nationalobesityforum.org.uk

British Dietetic Association
5th Floor, Charles House
148/9 Great Charles Street
Queensway
Birmingham
B3 3HT
Tel: 0121 200 8080
www.bda.uk.com

understanding food labels

The information provided by food labels can help you to select healthier food options. The labelling on food products provides nutritional information describing the product, where it comes from, and any processes it may have been through. The weight or volume is stated, and the ingredients are listed in descending order of content i.e. from the most to the least in the product. 'Use by' and 'sell by' dates are included, and foods which may cause allergic reactions in some people (milk, soya, nuts, gluten, eggs, etc.) are also often listed.

> Government legislation on food labelling exists to protect consumers against the ingredients on food products. Nutrition information is not required by law at present, but most manufacturers provide it voluntarily for customers. There are voluntary guidelines for nutrition claims that most manufacturers adhere to at present. The Food Standards Agency is presently consulting on proposals for new legislation and changes should become law in 2006. Labelling needs to be clear, concise, easy to understand and not misleading. A comprehensive list of food allergens will also be included to assist people with food allergies.

The nutritional information is then listed in a standard format starting off with the total energy per 100 g or 100 ml and the

quantities of each component per 100 g or 100 ml. Many
manufacturers also provide information for a serving, which
is helpful.

The components listed are as follows:

Energy (kJ and kcals)
Protein (g)
Carbohydrate (g)
of which sugars (g)
starches (g)
Fat (g)
of which saturates (g)
Polyunsaturates (g)
Monounsaturates (g)
Fibre (g)
Sodium (g)

> In order to convert sodium to the equivalent salt (sodium
> chloride), multiply by 2.5.

Manufacturers sometimes specify the total energy, protein,
carbohydrate and fat content of a product and other ingredients.

Products that claim to have a 'reduced' content e.g. fat or
sugar, must have at least 25% less of this component than the
standard product. Examples include low fat yoghurts or low sugar
desserts. Be aware, however, that some 'reduced fat' foods,
although having a reduced fat content compared with the standard
product, may still be high in fat., for example, crisps.

The following guide is useful when reading nutrition
information on labels.

THIS IS A LOT	THIS IS A LITTLE
(per 100 g food)	(per 100 g food)
20 g fat or more	3 g fat or less
5 g saturates or more	1 g saturates or less
0.5 g sodium or more	0.1 g sodium or less
10 g sugars or more	2 g sugars or less

When selecting foods in line with healthy eating guidance, you should choose foods that have less than:

- 10 g of fat per 100 g
- 10 g of sugar per 100 g for food and 2 g of sugar per 100 ml for drinks
- 0.5 g per 100 g of sodium (salt)

Guideline daily amounts (GDA) can also be found on some food labels. The figures are based on the requirements for an average adult of normal weight following a healthy diet. Values may be given for energy, fat, sugars and salt. These quantities are as follows.

Each day	Women	Men
Calories	up to 2000	up to 2500
Fat	up to 70 g	up to 95 g
Sugars	up to 50 g	up to 70 g
Salt	no more than 6 g	no more than 6 g

At present, there are voluntary guidelines for health claims. Such claims can include information like eating a food can improve health e.g. cholesterol lowering claims on spreads, healthy heart

Some manufacturers have their own logos for foods to indicate products that may be lower in either fat, sugar or salt. This can help you to choose a healthier option than the standard version of a particular food.

claims on oily fish products and healthy gut claims on bio-
yoghurts and probiotic drinks. These claims will be legislated once
the new laws regarding food labelling become statutory.

FOOD SAFETY

'Use by' dates are found on the labels of foods that perish easily.
Additionally these types of food will contain storage instructions.
Storage instructions must be adhered to if foods are to be safe to
eat within their 'use by' dates. A typical storage instruction is to
keep the food refrigerated at a temperature between 0 to 5°C.
Examples of foods which perish easily are milk, soft cheeses,
meats, ready prepared salads.

'Best before' dates are on the labels of foods that have a
longer shelf life. After the 'best before' date the product may begin
to lose its flavour or texture. Examples of these types of food
include frozen, canned and dried foods.

> To avoid the risk of food poisoning, follow instructions for
> food preparation and cooking carefully. Previously cooked
> food must be thoroughly reheated before eating, and
> cooked food should not be kept for more than two days
> unless you freeze it. You should never reheat food more
> than once.

glossary of ingredients

Bajhias/pakoras – onions, potatoes or mixed vegetables coated with gram flour and deep fried

Cardamom – aromatic spice – small green pods containing black seeds

Chapatti/roti – flat bread made with wheat flour, cooked in a pan

Chevda – Bombay mix, deep fried savoury snack made with split gram dahl, potato crisps, nuts and flaked rice

Cinnamon – aromatic spice – available in 'stick' or powder

Clove – aromatic spice used mainly in meat and rice dishes

Coconut milk – sold in cans; full fat and reduced fat versions available

Coriander – fragrant, green herb. Widely used in dishes and as a garnish

Coriander seeds – sweetly spiced beige seeds

Cumin – mild-flavoured sweet spice. Used as seeds and ground

Curry powder – spice mixture containing up to 20 spices

Dhal – lentil curry

Fennel seeds – green seeds with an anise-like flavour

Fenugreek seeds – yellowish seeds with a musky aroma

Garam masala – powder of mixed spices with cinnamon, black cardamom, black pepper, binger, cloves, coriander, cumin and red chillies

Garlic – important ingredient in many meat dishes

Ghee – clarified butter with a nutty taste

Ginger – rhizome with a sharp, pungent, cleansing taste

Halva – plain flour or semolina cooked with sugar and oil/ghee

Khir – Indian rice pudding

Masoor – red lentils

Methi – fenugreek

Mung dhal – green lentils

Mustard seeds – white (yellow in colour), brown and black varieties. Pungent when crushed, nutty and sweet when fried whole in oil

Nan – flat bread

Nutmeg – the dried seed of a pear-like fruit. Warm, sweet flavour

Raita – savoury yoghurt with cucumber, onion and/or tomatoes

Rice – many varieties are available. The aromatic, long grain Basmati rice has the lowest GI value

Samosas – triangular shaped pastry filled with minced meat or vegetables and deep fried

Sev – deep-fried savoury snack (like vermicelli) made with gram flour

Theplas – shallow-fried spiced chapatti made with wholemeal, gram and millet flours

Turmeric – dried, powdered spice, bright yellow in colour and musky aroma

index

Adam Daykin, PhD, BSc (Hons), MBA

Adam is an Intellectual Property Manager at NHS Innovations London. He has a PhD in Science and a Masters in Business Management (MBA). As an academic he authored 28 technical publications. Over the last 7 years he has specialised in developing novel innovations from initial concept through to commercial product.

Anne Claydon RGN

Lead Diabetes Nurse Newham University Hospital NHS Trust
Anne Claydon has been a Registered Nurse for over twenty years and an inpatient Diabetes Specialist Nurse for eight years. She is currently completing her MSc in Diabetes Care at Brighton University and is a member of the National Inpatient Nurse Forum.

Diana Markham, MA, BSc (Hons), Dip. Diet., Dip ADP

Chief Dietitian, Newham University Hospital NHS Trust
Diana is the Nutrition and Dietetic Services Manager at Newham University Hospital NHS Trust and has over 20 years experience working as a Dietitian in the NHS. She is a member of the British Dietetic Association (BDA).

Graham Toms MD FRCP

Consultant Physician and Endocrinologist, Newham University Hospitals NHS Trust
Graham became an NHS consultant specialising in diabetes in 1991. He has run the London Marathon six times between 1994 and 2004 and hopes there may one or two more to go. His dog is one of the fittest in East London.